Ethics in professional life

Ethics in professional life

virtues for health and social care

Sarah Banks
Ann Gallagher

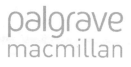

First published 2009 by
PALGRAVE MACMILLAN

Palgrave Macmillan in the UK is an imprint of Macmillan Publishers Limited,
registered in England, company number 785998, of Houndmills, Basingstoke,
Hampshire RG21 6XS.

Palgrave Macmillan in the US is a division of St Martin's Press LLC,
175 Fifth Avenue, New York, NY 10010.

Palgrave Macmillan is the global academic imprint of the above companies
and has companies and representatives throughout the world.

Palgrave® and Macmillan® are registered trademarks in the United States,
the United Kingdom, Europe and other countries.

ISBN-13: 978–0–230–50719–7
ISBN-10: 0–230–50719–0

This book is printed on paper suitable for recycling and made from fully
managed and sustained forest sources. Logging, pulping and manufacturing
processes are expected to conform to the environmental regulations of the
country of origin.

A catalogue record for this book is available from the British Library.

Library of Congress Cataloging-in-Publication Data
Banks, Sarah.
   Ethics in professional life : virtues for health and social care/Sarah Banks,
   Ann Gallagher.
      p. ; cm.
   Includes bibliographical references and index.
   ISBN-13: 978–0–230–50719–7
   ISBN-10: 0–230–50719–0
   1. Nursing ethics.   2. Professional ethics.   I. Gallagher, Ann, RGN.
   II. Title.
   [DNLM: 1. Ethics, Professional.   2. Ethics, Nursing.   3. Social Work—ethics.
   4. Virtues. W 50 B218e 2009]
   RT85.B36 2009
   174.2'9073—dc22   2008037815

10   9   8   7   6   5   4   3   2   1
18   17   16   15   14   13   12   11   10   09

Printed and bound in China

Contents

List of tables

List of vignettes

This book has been an exciting and challenging project. We have not only come to the project from two different practice disciplines (social work and nursing), but have had to work out ways of developing ideas, theories and approaches from a third discipline (moral philosophy) on the theme of virtue ethics.

The book could be described as 'hybrid' in more ways than one. The language of moral philosophical virtue theory (largely Aristotelian or neo-Aristotelian) is mixed with some of the more sociologically oriented practice theory of nursing and social work. The shared enterprise of writing has been a process of discovery and negotiation, not only between authors from two professional disciplines, with different types of experience, but also, we discovered, sometimes with rather different philosophical outlooks.

Ann Gallagher trained as a general and mental health nurse. She then studied philosophy and health studies at undergraduate level and medical and social ethics at Masters level. A doctorate in professional ethics (Gallagher, 2003) provided the opportunity to begin to explore the implications of virtue ethics for the professions. She is inclined towards a moderate neo-Aristotelian version of virtue ethical theory. This entails a focus on the virtues (dispositions towards promoting human flourishing) as central to understanding the moral life, with other features (duties, rights, principles and consequences of actions) regarded as necessary but secondary to virtues. She is interested in the relationship between empirical research and philosophical analysis, in the practice implications of concepts such as dignity and in explanations of unethical practice.

Sarah Banks studied mental philosophy at undergraduate level, completed a doctorate in social history, then worked as a community development officer and qualified as a social worker. She has a more pluralist view of ethics, viewing virtue ethics as one among several equally important and useful theoretical approaches to understanding and prescribing moral commitments and actions.

She is particularly interested in moral concepts such as 'integrity', 'care' and 'trustworthiness' as relations between people and in how these qualities are communicated as plausible and credible practice performances. She is also concerned about the way the political, policy and organisational contexts of practice create and constrain professional ethics as a study and a practice.

Our distinctive experiences and different perspectives have made the project of writing together both challenging and rewarding. It has meant some compromises in what we can claim in the book and may result in some (apparent) inconsistencies. One compromise is to present virtue ethics as one part of a framework for exploring and theorising important features of ethical life, rather than as a foundational ethical theory.

We both have gained enormously from this collaboration, learning from each other new arguments and ways of looking at practice, as well as what makes for good (or good enough) collaboration. We offer this book, the product of our first collaboration, to our readers in the hope that it goes some way towards meeting the aims we outline in the Introduction, and in the hope of developing the ideas through further dialogue between ourselves and others.

SARAH BANKS
Durham

ANN GALLAGHER
Kingston
May 2008

Acknowledgements

Many people have given help and support to us in the process of planning and writing this book. We are particularly grateful to all the practitioners upon whose interviews we have based many of the vignettes that are a vital part of the chapters on specific virtues. They were not only willing to give up their time, but also offered extremely thoughtful and thought-provoking accounts of and reflections on their practice and on the nature of their professions more generally. Our ideas have often been based on or developed from these reflections, without which the book would not have been possible. All accounts have been anonymised, with names of participants changed, in order to preserve the confidentiality of practitioners, service users, patients, family members and institutions. So we are not able to name individual interviewees, but do wish to express our sincere thanks for their generosity. Three of the vignettes are based on interviews conducted by Cynthia Bisman, to whom we are very grateful for the use of the material. Several vignettes are based on material from published reports and books, and we are grateful to the publishers for giving permission to use this material. We would also like to thank the three anonymous reviewers, who made helpful comments on the draft manuscript, enabling us to make improvements and clarifications.

We have benefited greatly from the support of our own institutions, Durham University and Kingston University & St George's University of London, which enabled us to arrange our work to allow extra time to complete the book in late 2007/early 2008. Sarah Banks is also grateful to the Centre for Research in Arts, Social Sciences and Humanities (CRASSH) at Cambridge University and Wolfson College for a very productive research fellowship in Autumn 2005 during which she undertook research on professional integrity; to the Institute of Advanced Study, Durham University for a Knott-Christopherson Fellowship and to Bryn Mawr College, USA, for a visiting scholarship in April 2008 (organised by Cynthia Bisman), that came at the time when the book needed to be revised, providing a stimulating and pleasant environment in which to work on the final version of the manuscript. Sarah Banks would also like to acknowledge the numerous conversations with colleagues in Durham and elsewhere that have helped develop her thinking in the field of ethics in professional life, including Cynthia Bisman, Hugh Butcher, Derek Clifford, Paul Hoggett, Richard Hugman, Tony Jeffs, Anne Marron, Marj Mayo, Chris Miller, Jean Spence, Robin Williams, the members of the European Social Ethics Project, the International Federation of Social Workers working group on ethics and numerous cohorts of community and youth work and social work students at Durham University whose practice dilemmas and reflective discussions are an eternal source of stimulation.

Ann Gallagher would like to acknowledge the generosity of Paul Wainwright in discussing and commenting on work in progress. She would like to express her gratitude to Ruth Chadwick, her PhD supervisor, who provided advice, encouragement and insights integrating ethical theory and everyday professional practice. Thanks are also owed to Joan McCarthy and Ian Byford who read and commented on draft chapters. Derek Sellman, Chris Belshaw, Chris Gastmans and Bob Brecher deserve acknowledgment for many thought-provoking and challenging conversations regarding virtue ethics and related issues. Other people who deserve a special mention for enhancing her understanding of the good life are her parents Raymond and Mary Margaret Gallagher, other family members, students, friends and colleagues – Brenda and Peter West, Liz and Tim Owen, Theresa Drought, Robert Stanley, Bill Burton, Jean McHale, Pat Lidiard, Verena Tschudin and Anne Davis to name a few. Most particularly, Ann would like to thank her daughter Kiera who endured disruption, during the development of the book, with patience and good humour.

We would also like to acknowledge the role played in the early stages of preparing the book proposal and finding a publisher by the late Jo Campling, and to express our gratitude to Lynda Thompson, Sarah Lodge and Kate Llewellyn at Palgrave Macmillan for their very positive encouragement and support.

The authors and publishers wish to acknowledge the article by Sarah Banks (2004), 'Professional Integrity, Social Work and the Ethics of Distrust', *Social Work and Social Sciences Review*, Vol. 11(2), published by Whiting & Birch, as an influence on the ideas and concepts addressed in Chapter 10 of this book; and the article by Ann Gallagher (2007), 'The Respectful Nurse', *Nursing Ethics*, Vol. 13(3), published by Sage as the basis for some of the discussion in Chapter 6.

Every effort has been made to trace all the copyright holders but if any have been inadvertently overlooked the publishers will be happy to make the necessary arrangements at the first opportunity.

Introduction

> To venture to write about the virtues is to subject one's
> self-esteem to constant bruising, to be made acutely aware,
> again and again, of one's own mediocrity. Every virtue is
> a summit between two vices, a crest between two chasms:
> hence courage stands between cowardice and temerity, dig-
> nity between servility and selfishness, gentleness between
> anger and apathy, and so on. But who can dwell on the high
> summits all the time? To think about the virtues is to take
> measure of the distance separating us from them. To think
> about their excellence is to think about our own inadequa-
> cies or wretchedness [...]. This treatise on the virtues will be
> useful only to those lacking in them.
>
> (Comte-Sponville, 2003, p. 5)

The main purpose of this book is to explore the nature and practice
of some of the moral qualities or 'virtues' regarded as important
for professional practitioners in the fields of health and social care.
We do this within the framework of a 'virtue-based' approach to
professional ethics, examining in turn the nature of several relevant virtues. The chosen virtues are professional wisdom, care,
respectfulness, trustworthiness, justice, courage and integrity.
Our approach could, perhaps, more accurately be described as
'virtues-based' or even 'virtues-oriented', signifying the book's
main focus on examining a range of virtues in professional life,
rather than exploring, developing or defending a virtue ethical
theory *per se* for health and social care. This brief introduction
describes the rationale for the book, its particular focus on nursing and social work, the nature of these two professional groups,
the relevance of virtues in professional life and an outline of the
book's content.

The rationale for the book

Our inspiration has come from the growing interest in virtue ethics amongst moral philosophers, which is slowly percolating through to professional ethics. As yet, however, there are few articulations of a virtue-based approach for the caring professions that offer detailed accounts of specific virtues from a practice perspective. We hope this book will play a part in developing the literature on the role of virtues in professional life, as well as helping practitioners think through what it means to be a good professional in the context of the many ethical complexities in contemporary health and social care work. Finally, by focusing primarily on two core professional groups, nursing and social work, we hope to encourage greater knowledge of each other's worlds and an increased readiness for the growing demands of inter-professional working in the fields of health and social care.

We believe the book is timely for a number of reasons. First, as indicated above, there has been a growing interest in virtue-based ethics in moral philosophy over the last 50 years, and this has trans-ferred more recently to professional ethics. Whilst some literature is emerging in the professional field, there are few book-length studies that focus on the analysis and practice of specific virtues (as opposed to applying or developing an ethical theory based on the virtues). Secondly, far-reaching changes are taking place in the organisation and practice of professional groups, including those involved in health and social care. In particular, the growth of inter-agency, inter-professional and integrated ways of working; the push to involve the public and service users in making decisions about needs and priorities; and the re-designation of 'patients' and 'clients' as customers and consumers present challenges to the power and distinctive value bases of existing professional groups. This is an opportune time, therefore, to examine a virtue-based approach to ethical values in the fields of health and social care. Thirdly, other shifts in the policy and organisational context are resulting in the marketisation of care, greater performance management and an intensification of systems of regulation of professional practitioners and the activities they perform. This seems to threaten key features of professional ethics, with the prospect of replacing ethical reflec-tion with professional regulation; professional judgement with standardised assessment and trusting relationships with contracts for care. A virtue-based approach to professional ethics shifts the focus onto the professional practitioners themselves: the kinds of people they are and could or should become, their commitments and competences and their roles as public service professionals.

Professional practitioners in health and social care, with particular reference to nursing and social work in Britain

The focus of this book is on professional health and social care practitioners. This potentially covers many different occupations, and we believe much of our discussion is relevant to a variety of professional practitioners (from doctors and occupational therapists to community development officers and childcare workers). However, in order to give the book a more defined focus, especially when discussing practice issues, we have placed a particular emphasis on nursing and social work. In the chapters on specific virtues where we use vignettes, the practitioners featured are more commonly nurses and social workers, although we have included some cases from other related professionals including midwives, a paramedic, a physiotherapist and a youth worker. Two of the vignettes are from the perspectives of service users.

Our practice examples are largely drawn from the British context, with one case from Ireland. We believe the subject matter of this book is relevant to practice in a range of countries, as many of the virtues are recognised worldwide. Indeed, nursing and social work are regarded as international professions. Each has international professional associations with statements on ethics that outline the values to which professionals should be committed worldwide. The extent to which the concept of internationally recognised and accepted values makes sense and/or is acceptable in reality is a subject of intense debate. The interesting fact remains that there are such international statements, which function at a kind of 'manifesto' level and attempt to draw together practitioners in quasi-social movements for improving health, social care and social justice across the world. However, insofar as virtues are developed and manifested in response to the particularities of situations (for example, being courageous by challenging bad practice in the workplace) and grounded in what some have argued are culturally relative concepts of what counts as the good life or human flourishing (for example, the valuing of freedom of speech and the minimisation of human suffering), then our analysis and discussion is firmly located in the context of current professional practice in Britain.

Social work

The institutional organisation and daily practice of both social work and nursing varies greatly across the world, as well as within different settings in one country. Social work is a particularly contested profession, with different practitioners and academics giving varying accounts of its purpose and role in society, depending upon their ideological positions, geographical and institutional locations. International definitions and statements of values tend to focus, therefore, on fairly general and abstract statements about role, purpose and methods. Nevertheless, such statements do provide a useful framework for identifying the broad purposes and boundaries of a profession. The definition offered by the International Federation of Social Workers (IFSW, 2000) is outlined below:

> The social work profession promotes social change, problem solving in human relationships and the empowerment and liberation of people to enhance well-being. Utilising theories of human behaviour and social systems, social work intervenes at points where people interact with their environments. Principles of human rights and social justice are fundamental to social work.

The purposes of social work are framed in terms of 'social change', 'empowerment' and 'liberation'. These terms indicate that social work as an international profession and social movement aspires to a purpose that is about more than just helping people to adapt to their environments. It is about enabling them to take action for themselves. The fact that the definition explicitly refers to principles of human rights and social justice as fundamental highlights the importance of social workers having a commitment to a set of core values. The mention of 'human rights' and 'social justice' covers both issues of individual freedom of choice and action and the distribution of power and resources in society.

The IFSW definition is followed by a commentary, which includes a fuller description of social work practice, suggesting that 'interventions range from primarily person-focused psychosocial processes to involvement in social policy, planning and development'. It is important to note that some of the activities that form part of these interventions (such as counselling or helping people obtain services and resources in the community) may be carried out by people who are not social workers (volunteers, family members, other welfare professionals). However, the location of the interventions undertaken by social workers within a rubric of theory and specialised terminology indicates that the practices will only be recognised as social work if they can be constructed in this way.

Although this international definition is useful as an attempt to unify those involved in the profession and practice called 'social work' throughout the world, it does not capture the essentially contested nature of social work and the constantly shifting views of its purpose. This is succinctly encapsulated by Payne (2000, p. 225), who points out that the nature of social work emerges from a balance at any point in time (or, we might add, in a particular country) between different views of its purpose, which we have summarised as:

▶ Maintaining the existing social order and providing individuals with services as part of a network of social agencies (*an individualist-reformist view*).
▶ Helping people attain personal fulfilment and power over their lives, so they feel competent to take part in social life (*a reflexive-therapeutic view*).
▶ Stimulating social change, transforming society by promoting cooperation, mutual support, emancipation, empowerment (*a socialist-collectivist view*).

Nursing

Nursing is also a wide-ranging and no less contested profession. The development of new roles within health care means that nurses are expanding the scope of their practice. Nurses engage in activities that were previously exclusively undertaken by doctors and other professionals. The renegotiation of the relationship between medicine and nursing has resulted in nurses becoming increasingly autonomous, transcending historical views of the role of the nurse as the doctor's 'handmaiden'. With the development of new roles (for example, clinical nurse specialists and nurse consultants), which require high levels of expertise and academic achievement, nurses are now in clinical leadership roles. Nurses work with people from cradle to grave and undertake a diverse range of interventions. They provide skilled intensive care to babies in neonatal care units, assist with surgery, provide talking treatments to people who experience mental distress, motivate and empower people in stroke rehabilitation units, provide palliative care towards the end of life, to name a few tasks and roles. Nursing practice continues to evolve, with nurses taking on new roles, resulting in a blurring of boundaries with other professions. Nurses may, for example, prescribe medication, perform diagnostic tests, make clinical diagnoses and refer people to other services. In some instances, nurses manage budgets and lead general practices and other health care organisations.

The diversity and complexity of nursing is suggested by the definition provided by the International Council of Nurses (2008):

> Nursing encompasses autonomous and collaborative care of individuals of all ages, families, groups and communities, sick or well and in all settings. Nursing includes the promotion of health, prevention of illness, and the care of ill, disabled and dying people. Advocacy, promotion of a safe environment, research, participation in shaping health policy and in patient and health systems management, and education are also key nursing roles.

In addition to the delivery of direct care, therefore, nurses also conduct research, work in management and education and shape health policy. The Royal College of Nursing (RCN, 2003) outlines the purpose of nursing as the promotion of growth, development, health and healing, and the prevention of illness and disease. The purpose of nursing is also, according to the RCN, to minimise suffering and distress, to enable people to understand and cope with disability and distress and to maintain quality of life until its end. The scope of nursing continues to expand with nurses gaining expertise in, for example, complementary therapy, surgical techniques and psychotherapeutic interventions. The development of the role of the nurse suggests challenges for the definition and purpose of nursing. Working in partnership with service users, carers and colleagues in other professions and agencies is necessary to achieve the purposes and ideals of nursing and of health and social care more broadly.

The virtues and professional life

The term 'virtue ethics' refers to a variety of ethical theories or theoretical approaches that have a central focus on the moral qualities ('virtues') of individual people and/or institutions. Virtue ethics has a long history in world philosophy and religion – commonly associated in Western philosophy with the fourth century BCE Greek thinker, Aristotle, but also featuring in the earlier writings of Confucius and in Buddhist, Christian and Islamic texts, for example. Although virtue ethics was the dominant form of ethical theorising in the ancient world, it was largely (although not completely) ignored in modern times, until its revival in Anglo-American philosophy from the mid-twentieth century.

While virtue ethics is becoming fashionable in the field of profes-, sional ethics, we are under no illusions that a virtue-based approach is easy to articulate or to justify in detail. The reasons for its theoretical appeal may also, paradoxically, be the same reasons why it is hard to implement in practice. Our current ways of organising, thinking about and doing professional work are dominated by concepts and practices of regulation, standardisation and contracts (based on notions of rights and obligations). It is partly as a reaction against this dominant paradigm that a virtue-based professional ethics seems attractive, with its focus on the individual professional as a moral agent within a community of practitioners who share a core moral purpose or 'service ideal'. However, as we shall discuss in Chapter 1, the notion of professions as communities of practitioners sharing a core moral purpose that is defined in terms of that practice (internal to it) is not straightforward either theoretically or in practice. For surely any profession's core purpose, if it still makes sense to say it has one, is grounded in broader societal (external) values. Furthermore, in practice, professions are fragmenting into specialist roles and tasks and integrating in super-teams where the notion of distinctive 'service ideals' may seem quaintly outmoded.

Outline of the book

As already indicated, this book takes what might loosely be described as a 'virtue-based' approach to professional ethics in the field of health and social care. This means that our focus of attention is primarily on the professional practitioners themselves: what kinds of moral qualities they exhibit and aspire to; how these are manifested in their professional commitments, relationships and actions; and how these qualities can be promoted and developed through professional practice and education. The nature and role of professional virtues is just one element of the theory and practice of professional ethics. Any complete picture of professional ethics would also take account of the nature and role of professional obligations and principles of right action; the nature of professional relationships with service users; the role of professions within society and the broader institutional and societal context of values and policies within which professional work is located. This book is, therefore, a partial account of professional ethics from a virtues perspective.

Chapter 1 explores the meanings of 'professional ethics' as a practice and as a subject of study. We argue that professional ethics is not reliant on an essentialist concept of professions as clearly demarcated occupational groups, although certain kinds of virtue-based approaches (based on notions of human flourishing) rely on the concept of a service ideal shared by members of a professional community. We examine the service ideals relevant to health and social care professions (restoring and maintaining health and social welfare).

In Chapter 2 we discuss the revival of interest in virtue ethics in moral philosophy and its relevance for professional ethics. We examine different varieties of virtue ethics and outline our own virtue-based approach, based on a notion of human flourishing, which is complementary to other theoretical approaches based on obligations, outcomes and relationships.

Chapter 3 explores the nature of virtues as excellent traits of character. We critically examine what is meant by 'character' and 'character traits', considering some of the challenges to the concept of character as comprising relatively stable and enduring dispositions. This chapter explores different classifications of virtues, the 'doctrine of the mean' and the nature of the 'emotion work' that goes into being virtuous in professional life. The chapter ends by outlining the rationale for our selection of virtues for further study in this book.

Chapters 4–10 explore specific virtues (professional wisdom, respectfulness, care, trustworthiness, justice, courage and integrity) in relation to the practice of health and social care professionals. The choice of these particular virtues (discussed in more detail in Chapter 3) reflects those we thought important and worthy of further elaboration. This list is by no means comprehensive, nor do we claim to have included just the most pertinent virtues. There are any number of other virtues that are equally applicable and important for the practice of health and social care that we have not included, as is demonstrated in the summary of different lists of virtues included in the Appendix to this book. For example, truthfulness is very important in both professional and personal life, and appears in some lists of professional virtues, while honesty features in other accounts. We have featured trustworthiness, but not honesty or truthfulness, as we judge they involve quite similar (although not the same) dispositions (related to reliability, doing what one has promised, not letting people down). Similarly, beneficence (Oakley and Cocking, 2001), benevolence (Beauchamp and Childress, 2001) or compassion (Beauchamp and Childress, 2001; Rhodes, 1986) might have been included. While these are not the same as care, which we have included, they do have some features in common in that they have concern for others as a central focus. Justice might have been framed as 'fairness', but we prefer 'justice' as a more all-embracing concept embodying elements of recognition of differences between people and groups, as well as fair distribution of goods and harms. What some theorists have called 'structural' or 'organising' virtues, namely, wisdom (specified as professional wisdom), courage and integrity, feature in many lists of generic and professional virtues and seem to us to be crucial in developing a virtue-based account of ethics in professional life. In short, the choice of virtues was arrived at on the basis of what we felt a rounded picture of professional life might require, including moral dispositions relating to recognising, forming and sustaining relationships with service users and others; giving and distributing goods; making good judgements; and challenging incompetent, discriminatory and oppressive norms, institutions and practices. Within this framework we chose particular virtue concepts that we felt interested in and/or competent to write about.

Each chapter starts with several vignettes describing aspects of practice in health and social care. Many of these are based on interviews with practitioners conducted for this book, or for previous research projects, while some are drawn from the reports of professional bodies, public inquiries or the work of other authors. All relate to real situations, albeit suitably anonymised. Our reason for starting our discussions of the virtues in this way is to ground the chapters in practice. We are privileged to have had access to the

perspectives of practitioners and service users regarding their experiences of ethical practice. In the interviews we conducted sometimes practitioners spoke explicitly about their understanding of,
and commitment to, specific virtues. At other times, they talked
more generally about what they valued and their experience of ethically challenging situations. The process of selecting and abstracting
from the material we had, then writing and reflecting on the individual vignettes was, for us, challenging. At times, it felt like a process of excavation. We felt like ethicist–practitioner–archaeologists,
not quite sure what we were looking for, nor how to make sense of
what we found; also afraid of digging too deep and damaging the
integrity of a person or their story. We were aware of the limitations
of the accounts we had, which although rich and diverse, were but
remnants of complex narratives. We were also aware of our own
limitations, feeling sometimes that it was somewhat audacious to
position ourselves as people sufficiently wise to extract key mes-
sages from practice vignettes. It is not our view, however, that the
last word has been said on any of the virtues or vignettes discussed
but rather it is our hope that these chapters will provoke thought
and dialogue.

After brief analytical reflections on the vignettes, these chapters
then move into a conceptual analysis of the chosen virtues, examining different meanings and interpretations of the virtue concepts,
and linking these, where appropriate, to the vignettes. Each chapter ends with a consideration of possible strategies for practice and
professional education that might help develop and sustain these
virtues in professional life.

In the conclusion, we reflect on the value of taking a situated
virtue-based perspective on ethics in professional life and explore
the inter-professional potential of a virtue-based approach.

Chapter 1

The domain of professional ethics

Introduction

In this chapter we examine different meanings of 'professional ethics' in practice and as a subject of study, considering the extent to which the concept of 'profession' still makes sense in the current climate of occupational restructuring and increasing state regulation. We suggest that the rationale for professional ethics in practice derives to a large extent from the conditions of vulnerability, dependence and power in which professional practice takes place, especially in the fields of health and social care. We then explore the nature and function of professional service ideals in grounding professional ethics in the intrinsically valued goods of repairing and maintaining health and social welfare.

A preview: vignettes from practice

The subject matter of this book is ethics in professional life, with a focus on the feelings, thoughts and actions of professional practitioners in the context of their work. The following short accounts are summaries of some of the vignettes discussed in the chapters on specific moral qualities of professional practitioners in health and social care. Most of the vignettes are either written from the perspective of professional practitioners or have a focus on the attitudes, activities and accomplishments of professional practitioners in the context of their relationships with service users, family members, students, other professionals and professional bodies.

1. A nursing student observes a qualified nurse passing a naso-gastric tube (a tube going through the nose to the stomach in order to drain the stomach) on a woman diagnosed with cancer. The student notices the nurse's *patience and sense of humour* as he gains the co-operation and *trust* of the woman.

2. A senior social worker describes supervising a student who is working with a Sikh young man described as having moderate learning difficulties and mental health problems. Police had recently arrested the young man for chasing and possibly assaulting two young women in a park. The social worker feels the young man is facing discrimination on the grounds of his religion and ethnicity, his intellectual abilities and his mental health. The social worker is supporting the student in taking on *the role of advocate* on behalf of the Sikh family.

3. Midwives draw attention to the unacceptable practices of an obstetrician. The inquiry team examining the case states that they 'had difficulty understanding why so few had the *courage, insight, curiosity or integrity* to say: "This is not right"'.

4. A social worker attends a school consultation meeting where children giving cause for concern are discussed. When she asks about the progress of one of the children, a teacher describes the child's mother as 'a waster, she's such a complete drug addict'. The social worker sees this as *disrespectful* and challenges the teacher, who then apologises.

5. A nurse is removed from the professional register of qualified nurses and midwives for falsifying research data. The professional conduct committee hearing the case refers to the nurse's *dishonesty and breach of trust.*

6. A service user with learning disabilities describes her relationship with a social worker, commenting that she was 'the first one who was interested [. . .] she really knew what she was doing, *I trusted her.* She has always given me the right advice [. . .]. It feels good knowing that she is there for me.'

7. A physiotherapist describes the *wisdom* of a senior colleague who always seems to know the right question to ask.

8. A paramedic describes her *fear* as she approaches a mother holding a child who appears dead.

These examples were selected because they provide insights into the qualities of the good professional and give accounts of instances of ethical lapses or situations where professionals reacted to the behaviour of others. It is these kinds of dispositions, situations, processes and relationships that form an important part of the subject matter of professional ethics and on which we hope to shed some light in the course of the book.

What is missing from these brief vignettes is, of course, the broader contexts in which the scenarios are located. These would include further details of the biographies and identities of professional and service user participants (such as life histories, types of professional/service user experience, ethnicity, gender, class and age), the nature and purposes of the organisation for which the practitioners work, the lines of power and accountability, the political, legal and policy contexts. This is one of the dangers of using vignettes – they encourage us to focus attention on one particular situation or incident isolated in time and place. We have tried to include in our longer versions of these vignettes in later chapters as much as we can about the emotions, thoughts or reflections of the people (mainly professionals) whose stories are told, as this is the focus of our concern in writing about virtue ethics. However, the danger of a focus on the individual professional practitioners involved is that the perspectives of service users, the organisational constraints, structural inequalities and societal pressures that greatly influence professional work are left in the background. We will reflect further on this common criticism of virtue ethics in later chapters and at the end of the book.

The nature of professional ethics

As the title indicates, we have located this book within the realm of professional ethics. The term 'professional ethics' has many connotations and is partly influenced by how we define 'professional' and 'ethics'.

'Professions' and 'professional'

One way of understanding the adjective 'professional' is to take it to refer to the activities and approaches of those occupations that can be categorised as 'professions'. There are, however, different interpretations of what counts as a 'profession'. Some writers on professional ethics view 'professions' quite narrowly as occupations that have certain traits, such as a code of ethics, a service ideal, specialist education and expertise and a degree of occupational control over membership and standards (see, for example, Airaksinen, 1998). This traditional trait-based approach might result in medicine and law, for example, being regarded as full professions; nursing, social work and engineering as semi-, aspirant or pseudo-professions; and child-minding or refuse collection as non-professions. An alternative perspective is to see 'professions' more broadly as occupational groups that make bids for certain kinds of status and power and/or that may move along different trajectories according to conditions pertaining in different countries and different time periods (Johnson, 1972; Siegrist, 1994).

The first view of professions can be categorised as relatively narrow and essentialist, entailing that an occupational group only counts as a profession if it possesses certain key characteristics. The alternative view takes a more historical and developmental perspective, studying changing structures of power, status, control and organisation within occupational groups and between these occupations and the broader society of which they are a part. While the essentialist approach has largely been superseded in sociological accounts of the professions, it persists in some of the philosophical literature on professional ethics, including virtue-based approaches. So although we do not think that the essentialist view of professions has much purchase in the study of the practice of professional groups, it may be required, if only as an 'ideal type' to ground some virtue-based accounts of professional ethics. We will return to this point later in this chapter.

In this book, we do not focus much attention on the debates about what counts as a 'profession', since we interpret the term 'professional' more broadly than simply 'pertaining to professions as identifiable occupational groups'. We regard the adjective 'professional' as being about the roles people play, relationships they conduct and activities they perform in the course of their work in the context of some kind of occupational structure. The occupational structure may take the form of a traditional professional structure as defined by the trait theorists, but it may also take a much looser form – with occupational groups constantly in a process of forming and reforming, with permeable and overlapping boundaries.

If we just take the example of occupations in the welfare and caring field in Britain in recent decades, we can get a picture of the complexity of current practice. We can see a simultaneous process of 'professionalisation' of specific occupational groups, at the same time as there has been and is a clustering together and state-initiated standardisation of their practices. For example, new groupings have formed around particular types of work, developing their own professional or occupational associations and standards (for example in complementary therapy, counselling, youth work and community development work). Yet at the same time, state regulation of the work of these and all occupational groups has also proceeded, involving a huge national enterprise of defining occupational standards (taking into account the needs of employers, service users, and national social and economic priorities). The increasing emphasis on the role of service user groups in the defining and monitoring of occupational standards in practice and educational contexts is particularly noteworthy. In the case of the larger and more established occupational groups, there has also been a process of reforming or initiating statutory regulatory bodies to oversee these standards, including keeping national registers of qualified professionals.

In the health care field in Britain, the Nursing and Midwifery Council (NMC) replaced the former UK Central Council for Nursing, Midwifery and Health Visiting in 2002. The Health Professions Council, set up in 2001, was recorded in 2007 as regulating 13 health professions including art therapists, chiropodists, dietitions, occupational therapists and physiotherapists. New regulatory bodies covering social work and a variety of types of 'social care work' were established in each country of Britain in 2001. All of these bodies cover more than one occupational group and set standards and monitor practice. They produce codes of ethical practice or conduct which, in some instances, sit alongside or seem to have almost superseded the ethical codes of the professional associations, of which membership is voluntary (such as the British Association of Social Workers).

Despite the challenges to the concept of identifiable professions, the idea of separate professions persists in professional literature and programmes of professional education and qualification. Although in Britain separate professions have been clustered together within occupational groupings for the purpose of developing standards and professional registration, their identities within professional education remain for the moment. Despite increasing trends towards inter-professional and integrated working in practice, and some programmes of inter-professional education, distinct professional identities are still available for practitioners as 'social worker', 'nurse', 'midwife' and so on. Yet at the same time there is no doubt that post-qualifying practice in inter-professional teams and projects may lead professionals into taking on a variety of roles perhaps once considered outside their profession's remit, and sub-scribing to team/role specific norms and values. So the situation is fluid and the question remains as to how strong the communities of practice are and can remain in the context of increasing consolidation and control from external institutional and statutory forces.

The example of these changes in the structures of occupational control in the fields of health and social care in Britain illustrates that in studying 'professions' or aspects of professional life, an historical/developmental approach is helpful. This entails seeing the concept of 'profession' as dynamic and shifting, taking into account a range of significant actors and stakeholders (including state, professions, professional organisations, professionals, service users, service user organisations, the media and public opinion).

'Ethics' and 'professional ethics'

The domain of 'ethics' is equally contested, depending upon what ethical theory is held, if any. Broadly speaking, we include within 'ethics' matters relating to the norms of right and wrong action, good and bad dispositions or 'character' traits and the nature of the good life. Whilst some theorists distinguish the domain of the 'ethical' (values concerning the nature of the good life, which may be culturally relative) from the domain of the 'moral' (concerning universal norms of right action), we use the two terms interchangeably in this book. It is important to note, however, that the term 'ethics' is itself used in two rather different ways in the English language: as a plural term denoting the actual values and norms people hold or follow (as in 'Jane's ethics are suspect') and as a singular term referring to the study of norms and values (as in 'Jane is studying ethics [moral philosophy] at university').

This then leads to two understandings of professional ethics:

1. *Professional ethics in practice*: the norms of right action, good qualities of character and values relating to the nature of the good life that are aspired to, espoused and enacted by professional practitioners in the context of their work.

2. *Professional ethics as a subject area*: the study of the norms of right action, good qualities of character and values relating to the nature of the good life that are aspired to, espoused and enacted by professional practitioners in the context of their work.

Professional ethics in this second sense, as the study of norms and values in professional practice, is usually regarded as part of an academic or professional discipline or subject area. Most commonly, professional ethics is seen as a sub-discipline or area of study within moral philosophy, often as a specialism of what is commonly called 'applied' or 'practical' ethics. However, it can be regarded equally as a specialist subject within a particular professional discipline (for example, social work ethics might be categorised as part of the discipline of social work). Whilst these distinctions may seem somewhat pedantic, they do help us understand the rather different approaches that can be found in the literature on professional ethics. The more philosophical literature often focuses either on applying an ethical theory to a professional field (for example, a duty-based approach to medical ethics) in order to test or elucidate the ethical theory or on conceptual analysis with the aim of clarifying arguments and removing confusion (for example, analysing different meanings of 'informed consent' and showing they are contradictory or incompatible). The more practice-based literature, on the other hand, tends to focus on the description and analysis of practical problems and dilemmas or on practitioners' value stances and beliefs, drawing on professionally recognised concepts (such as confidentiality, professional integrity, social control) and sometimes undertaking empirical studies based on methodologies from other social science disciplines such as sociology, anthropology or psychology.

In between these two approaches lies what might be termed a 'hybrid approach' that combines concepts and theoretical resources from both moral philosophy and professional practice disciplines (which themselves draw on the scientific, social scientific and arts disciplines). This is a challenging approach to take. It risks criticism from moral philosophers as 'amateur philosophy', over-simplification or sheer misguidedness. From practitioners and practitioner academics it risks incomprehension or criticism as irrelevant, overly abstract and out of touch with reality. So the hybrid approach, which is, in effect, what we do in this book, requires a degree of judgement about which of the philosophers' fine-grained distinctions and abstract debates are germane and helpful for understanding the practice context and which aspects of a particular theory or approach are not really transferable outside the world of moral philosophy. The terminology of moral philosophers when talking about a concept such as a 'virtue' (which may imply that a virtue is an entity with powers, a possession or an inner state) does not always fit easily with that of other disciplines (for example, a sociological discourse analysis approach might view virtues as dispositions or performances). This is a book that is essentially about making sense of practice, so our interests and motivations for the study are in the practice field. However, we do develop and draw on a largely moral philosophical account of virtues, modifying and adapting it to our own ends. There is, therefore, a symbiotic relationship between philosophical ideas and vignettes from everyday practice.

Vulnerability, dependency and power

'Vulnerability' is an important concept in ethics generally, and particularly in professional ethics. One of the commonly cited reasons for the need for professional ethics in practice (including written codes of ethics) is that professionals are especially powerful in relation to the users of their services, who are therefore vulnerable to exploitation, abuse or other forms of poor and inappropriate treatment. This is particularly apparent in the case of health and social care, where the users of professional services may be in states of poor health, material poverty, social need or crisis. Yet even in the cases where the service users may be healthy, rich and powerful (users of the services of private doctors, architects, barristers or accountants), the 'professionals' have power deriving from their special knowledge and expertise and perhaps their position as gatekeepers to other services or resources required by the 'clients' or service users. It is important, therefore, for professional practitioners to be very aware of the power inherent in their roles, the vulnerability of the people who use their services and the dependence that service users may have on the professionals.

Thinking of vulnerability in relation to the practice of health and social care, there is a tendency to see it as a concept associated with people who are sick or in social crisis and as negative (leaving people open to harm), yet as MacIntyre (1999) comments, as human beings we are all vulnerable to a range of afflictions at various times in our lives, and our survival and flourishing are in no small part owed to others. Vulnerability and dependency are therefore inevitable facts of the human condition. Furthermore, whilst vulnerability is associated with human fragility and fallibility, leaving us open to harm and mistakes, this very fragility is also associated with a more positive emotional openness, sensitivity and willingness to relate to others through loving and caring relationships. It is important not to lose sight of the positive aspects of vulnerability in professional relationships, while being equally aware of the potential for damage.

Sellman (2005) usefully distinguishes 'ordinary vulnerability' (applying to all humans) and 'more-than-ordinary vulnerability' (applying to those who are incapacitated in some way by, for example, disability or illness). Elaborating on this distinction he says:

> We are ordinarily vulnerable just so long as we retain the capacity to act in ways that offer us some protection against everyday harms. We are more-than-ordinarily vulnerable when, for whatever reason, we do not have that capacity. So our vulnerability is not merely a function of the extent of our exposure to harm but it is also a function of our capacity for self-protection.
>
> (Sellman, 2005, p. 5)

For people who are extraordinarily vulnerable, feeling vulnerable, that is, being aware of potential dangers and harms, can be a positive protection as it encourages them to limit their exposure to harm. This suggests that it may not always be appropriate for professional practitioners in caring roles to work to reduce people's sense of vulnerability. Professionals themselves will experience ordinary vulnerability, but may also become especially vulnerable in certain circumstances as they undertake their professional roles. In some situations, health and social care practitioners risk catching infectious diseases, experiencing violent attacks from service users or losing their reputations or jobs through making a wrong judgement. Furthermore, when caring for people who are dependent upon them for their health or well-being, professional practitioners themselves become vulnerable. Kittay (1999) makes this point in discussing unpaid, involuntary dependency workers (for example, mothers caring for their children). They are in a unique position to harm or benefit the other people, and this work itself carries a heavy moral load. Professional workers may be in a similar position, although with some degree of institutional and legal protection.

Arguably the most significant positive outcome of recognising and responding appropriately to vulnerability is human flourishing. The ability to respond appropriately to different types of vulnerability (physical, psychological, emotional, existential and ethical) is dependent on the vulnerable person's own characteristics – for example, on their resilience; on the willingness and ability of others to contribute to or thwart the person's flourishing; and on the nature of the institutions or environments inhabited by the parties involved (are they enabling or disabling?).

The ground of professional ethics: intrinsic goals and service ideals

Drawing on the above discussion, an important element of the rationale for professional ethics could be said to be the provision of a framework for professional relationships in contexts of vulnerability and dependency. Focusing particularly on the power of professionals and vulnerability of service users, it is essential that professionals have a commitment to work for the good of service users in the broader context of the public good. Taking into consideration also the burden of responsibility placed on health and social care professionals, who may find themselves in situations of varying degrees of risk, it also seems important that the roles they take on are actually contributing to a socially valued purpose. This leads to the notion of professions having a core purpose or service ideal that could be described as 'good in itself' underpinning their practices and recognised by professionals, service users and the general public.

Much of what has been written about professional ethics, especially from a virtue ethics perspective, is either explicitly or implicitly premised upon an essentialist view of professions. An assumption is made that there are relatively clearly defined professions with identifiable core purposes or service ideals. This is not to deny that norms and standards of practice and what counts as expertise are constantly evolving and disputed. This may include disputes, for example, about what counts as 'informed consent' and when it can or should be over-ridden; what is 'child abuse' and what is accepted as credible expertise in its identification. However, underlying all this, the argument goes, there is a relatively enduring core purpose or ideal at the heart of each profession that is recognised and lived out by the professionals in their practice. This is a social purpose that is recognised as a good for individuals, families and the wider community or society and is what gives the professions their legitimacy and grounds their professional ethics. For medicine and health care professions generally this has often been identified as the restoration and maintenance of 'health'. While there is less literature on this theme for social work and social care, the ideal of 'welfare' or 'social welfare' has been suggested for social work. This view of professional ethics is, perhaps, most clearly articulated in the work of Koehn (1994) in her book, *The Ground of Professional Ethics*. Her main focus is the examination of the moral legitimacy of the professional role. According to Koehn, what grounds professional ethics (as a set of norms, values and practices) is the pledge professionals make to serve some higher good – that is, a good that goes beyond their own self-interest, that focuses on the good of other individuals and ultimately the public good. These sorts of goods or ends of the professions are sometimes called service ideals, although Koehn herself does not use that term. They are regarded as good in themselves (that is, they are not a means to an end, such as individual wealth, group status or social control). In terms of the professions she is studying (medicine, law and the ministry), Koehn (1994, pp.70–71) identifies their good ends as health, legal justice and salvation. While these professions may have other ends or purposes (to provide individual fulfilment or an income for talented people who work as professionals; to sustain a physically and spiritually healthy workforce in order to maintain the economy and generate wealth), the main point is that one major component of the professions' ends is *an end desired for its own sake*. According to Oakley and Cocking (2001, p. 74) a good profession is one that involves a key commitment to a human good, a good that plays a crucial role in enabling us to live a flourishing life.

The idea of a service ideal has been characterised in the literature in several different ways by different authors using different terminology, but broadly referring to similar concepts: the *end* or *telos* of a profession; an *intrinsic goal or purpose*; a *service ideal*; or a *regulative ideal*. Critics have identified a number of problems with these ideas. Beauchamp (2003), for example, taking the case of medicine, argues that it is not possible to see it as having an intrinsic end. The concept of medicine is too ill-formed, he argues, and ordinary language, schools of medicine and legal definitions fail to provide exact boundaries. The same argument would clearly apply to all other professions. However, we could argue that the fact that there are practical difficulties in defining the boundaries of professions does not necessarily mean that the concept of a service ideal or intrinsic end is meaningless. This is only the case if we think the 'ideal' is linked very closely to the core purpose of a clearly identifiable professional group. The ideals identified above, namely health and welfare, are clearly shared by many related occupational groups.

Another criticism, however, relates to the question of whether we can really separate intrinsic (internal) and extrinsic (external) goods or ends in the way Koehn (1994, pp. 71–76) and others suggest. Surely, argues Beauchamp (2003, p. 32), physicians (and we might add nurses and social workers) can and do provide many important benefits to society and service users that are 'externally' defined – for example, reproductive controls and technologies, occupational health, crime prevention and safeguarding children. If we return to Koehn's account of health as an intrinsic good, she also acknowledges the fact that there are many externally defined goods of medicine of the type Beauchamp lists. The point she makes, however, is that 'at least one major component' of the professions' ends is an end desired for its own sake (Koehn, 1994, p. 71). That is, a profession and the professionals operating within it may have several goals, some of which may not be good in themselves (they may be extrinsic goods), but they must have at least one core intrinsic good at their heart.

Oakley and Cocking (2001, p. 87) make a similar point when they state that extrinsic goods, such as efficiency in resource allocation or respecting service users' autonomy, may also be regarded as goals of medicine (or in our case, nursing and social work). However, these should be regarded as 'side-constraints' rather than the core goals or guiding ideals of practice. A similar argument applies to the aims of individual practitioners for making money or achieving high status – if these were to become the overall guiding ideals or goals of practice, then arguably the practitioner would be a morally flawed occupant of the professional role.

Service ideals as regulative, rhetorical and aspirational

While there are some difficulties with the concept of a 'service ideal', it is important not to take the concept too literally. We might regard its function as an heuristic device (a model offering guidance), or an ideal type of what professional work might be at its best, rather than an accurate representation of what it currently is. Freidson (1983, p. 32), in his study of the professions, describes 'profession' itself as a 'folk concept', which has no single definition and 'no attempt at isolating its essence will ever be persuasive'. This analysis applies equally to the concept of the professional service ideal, which we could characterise as a myth, folk concept or rhetorical device. This does not mean that it is not in use and not useful. On the contrary, it performs a valuable role in guiding practitioners in striving and aspiring towards individually fulfilling and socially useful professional lives.

A slightly different variation of the service ideal as a 'regulative ideal' is offered by Oakley and Cocking (2001, pp. 25–31), which might help our appreciation of the nature of this rather contested concept. They present this concept in the course of developing a virtue ethical account of medicine and law. Their concept of a 'regulative ideal' is useful in two ways: it is framed in terms of how individual practitioners live out the 'ideal' in practice and it is very clear that the ideal goes beyond what is codified in extant codes of professional ethics. According to Oakley and Cocking (2001, p. 25):

> To say that an agent has a regulative ideal is to say that they have internalised a certain conception of correctness or excellence, in such a way that they are able to adjust their motivation and conduct so that it conforms – or at least does not conflict – with that standard.

On this account, regulative ideals are normative dispositions that may be general in scope or specific to certain parts of life or activities. In the case of professional life, part of being a good nurse or social worker would be to have internalised a conception of what the appropriate ends of nursing or social work are and to be disposed to treat service users in ways that are consistent with these ends. Oakley and Cocking (2001, p. 27) make the important point that regulative ideals can guide and govern professionals' action, without being one of their purposes or motives in acting. Their notion of a regulative ideal includes normative dispositions governing actions according to standards of correctness (that may be codifiable as principles and rules), and standards of excellence that go beyond the merely correct or incorrect (that are not codifiable).

'Health' and 'social welfare' as regulative ideals

Health

Koehn (1994, pp. 71–76) gives an account of 'health' as an intrinsic good in the context of medicine, later acknowledging that if nursing can be conceived of as having an intrinsic good, then this too would be 'health' (p. 179). If we take serving health to be the central goal of health care professions, then we need to explore in a little more detail what this entails. Koehn (1994, pp. 71–76) offers an account of health as 'wholeness'. She argues that living organisms possess an intrinsic wholeness manifested in their capacity to grow, develop and mature. They preserve a boundary between the inside and the outside of an organism and have some limited capacity to restore themselves to wholeness if damaged (for example, damaged skin tissue is replaced with new in animals; plants will regrow missing roots). As Koehn (1994, p. 72) comments,

> Being healthy seems to mean maintaining the whole. The unhealthy organism is one which has lost the ability to differentiate and maintain the whole with all of its parts.

However, health is more than just being whole, it is also a dynamic process. Koehn speaks of the need for the whole organism to engage in activity to keep individual parts functioning (for example, muscles waste if not used). This is about developing appropriate habits; Koehn describes this as 'well-habitedness', which affects the course of the life we lead. We can choose which habits to develop and whether to prioritise care of our bodies over and above other purposes or choices. This suggests that health involves a balance between inherited or acquired diseases or limitations and the use of our bodies in relation to our plans or desires. If we see health as the balanced functioning of a well-habited whole, argues Koehn, it is clear that it is good both from the perspective of the individual and the wider community. As Koehn (1994, p. 75) comments, 'Health, like life, is good in itself because health is the balanced striving (i.e. living) of an organism with a career. Where there is no health, living is attenuated'. Although this account focuses on bodily health, clearly it could and should be extended to include mental health, given the focus on 'wholeness'.

This account of health as 'wholeness' seems to be based on a particular view of human nature and the function of human beings as whole organisms whose end or *telos* is to achieve and/or maintain this organic wholeness. It is perhaps rather metaphorical and all-embracing and seems almost equivalent to 'flourishing' rather than simply a part of what contributes to human flourishing or well-being. Oakley and Cocking (2001, pp. 76), in attempting to give an account of 'health' that can function as the central goal of medicine, define it more specifically in terms of 'normal biological and psychological functioning'. By this they mean functioning at a level typical of human beings (of a particular sex, age group and so on). Even when patients cannot be healed or have their health restored, health professionals can serve health in many ways by helping patients to minimise various impairments to functioning or alleviating distressing symptoms. While Oakley and Cocking's account of health is more specific than that of Koehn, it raises a lot of questions about what counts as 'normal' and who defines 'normality'. The use of the concept 'normal' may lead to a devaluation of people with physical and mental states that fall outside the boundaries of 'normal' (for example, people experiencing mental distress, learning or physical disability such as schizophrenia, Down's Syndrome or amputation). For these reasons, Koehn's much broader account of health as wholeness, conceived of as wholeness for this human being, with this career and life course, is more satisfactory, if less specific only to medicine or health care. It leads very easily into the concept of human flourishing, which we will address in more detail in Chapter 2.

Social welfare[1]

Less has been explicitly written on the notion of a service ideal for the social care professions. Airaksinen (1994, p. 8) suggests in passing that 'welfare' is the service ideal for social work. This seems an even broader and more all-embracing concept than 'health'. Several social policy theorists examining this concept (for example, Brandt, 1976; Marshall, 1976) resort to dictionary definitions in a search for enlightenment. Here we find welfare defined as: 'Happiness, well-being, good health or fortune (of a person, community, etc)' (*The New Shorter Oxford English Dictionary*, 1993, p. 3653). This is surely too vague to serve as the core purpose of a profession. As the definition above suggests, the term 'welfare' embraces both individual welfare (the well-being of individual people) and social welfare (which may be regarded as the sum total of all individuals' welfare, or as some form of communal or collective well-being, not necessarily reducible to the sum of individuals' welfare). What is regarded as comprising welfare or well-being will vary between individuals and societies over time, but in this respect it is probably no more problematic as a concept than 'health'.

---

[1] Banks, S. (2004) *Ethics, Accountability and the Social Professions*, Basingstoke, Palgrave Macmillan, pp. 55–58.

Our use of the term 'welfare' in relation to the social care professions immediately has connotations of 'welfare state', given that many of the professionals work within or are at least mandated and controlled through the social and community services of the local and central state. Those aspects of well-being that are the business of the social care professions tend to be linked to mitigating the ill-effects of poverty, social exclusion, abusive behaviour, individual psychological and physical challenges and promoting community cohesion and democratic participation. This includes a concern with both individual and social welfare. While the individuals of day-to-day concern to most professionals are current service users, professionals also have a significant concern for potential service users, ordinary citizens and taxpayers. Hence 'welfare' includes an element of 'social control', both indirectly in its attempts to mitigate certain social problems at an individual level and more overtly in its work to prevent and challenge child abuse or youth offending, to create cohesive neighbourhoods or to prevent people from harming themselves and others in cases of mental ill health, for example.

However, is 'welfare' specific enough to fulfil the function of the core purpose of the social care professions? Clark (2000), in exploring the core purpose of social work, suggests that welfare is too broad and is shared with other parts of the welfare state. He suggests a more specific purpose as 'to promote the realisation of ordinary life' (Clark, 2000, p. 129). Social workers intervene when there is a discrepancy between the normative (moral) standards generally understood in a particular community and the actual conditions of ordinary life. This is still rather general, but as Clark points out, social work is committed to the indivisibility of welfare – that is, individual well-being encompasses safety, health, housing, financial security and so on. His characterisation of the core purpose is more specific than our dictionary definition of 'welfare'. For Clark's version locates well-being in a social context of commonly accepted standards of what counts as ordinary living. Like Koehn's account of health, this is a very holistic account of welfare. However, by explicitly defining welfare in relation to commonly understood standards of ordinary life in a particular community, this account is less 'naturalistic' than the holistic account of health, since it is not based on a semi-metaphysical account of what counts as a good (in the sense of well-functioning) community. We could interpret this account of welfare as implying that what counts as ordinary living may be disputed and will change over time (that is, it is subject to ongoing debate and revision within society and the community of professional practitioners). The emphasis on welfare in a social context also leads us to suggest that 'social welfare' might be a more appropriate characterisation of the service ideal of social work than simply 'welfare'.

Thus, we may conclude that if we had to identify a general all-embracing core purpose or service ideal for the social care professions comparable to those identified in much of the literature on professional ethics for medicine and law, then 'welfare' would fulfil this role. More specifically, this could be construed as 'social welfare', if we want to encapsulate the notion of the promotion of individual well-being in a social context as well as communal or collective well-being.

Concluding comments

Our discussion in this chapter suggests that the concept of identifiable professions with unique core purposes or service ideals does not fit neatly with many aspects of our current experience of professional life in Britain. However, it nevertheless seems possible to suggest that professionals working in health care share a common regulative ideal concerned with restoring and maintaining people's health, and those in social care professions share a core goal relating to the promotion of social welfare. Both these 'ends' are so general and relatively all-embracing that they overlap considerably with each other and encompass a large part of what we might see as human flourishing in general. This suggests that there may be considerable commonality at a general level in what counts as a good health care professional and as a good social care professional, even if the implementation of these ideals in practice differs according to the different circumstances of the work.

Chapter 2

Virtue ethics and professional life

Introduction

In modern moral philosophy and recent professional ethics, the question: 'what ought I to do?' has preoccupied philosophers and practitioners alike. That is, the main focus of attention has been the actions or conduct of the moral agent. This contrasts markedly with the focus in ancient classical and medieval moral philosophy and religion on the question 'how should I live?', referring to life both as an individual and within a society. In Anglo-American moral philosophy in the last five decades, however, there has been a revival of interest in this latter question, manifested in terms of a focus on the character of the moral agent, expressed in terms of virtues and vices, and theorised as virtue ethics. Virtue ethics has become a legitimate contender as an alternative, complementary or supplementary approach to obligation-based or consequentialist ethical theories. This chapter introduces virtue ethics and discusses the central tenets and potential of the approach for the health and social care professions.

Virtue theory and virtue ethics

Before discussing virtue ethics, it is important to distinguish 'virtue theory' from 'virtue ethics' (Driver, 1996, p. 111). The term 'virtue theory' is used to refer to accounts of the nature of virtues – what they are, what functions they perform and how they operate. Such accounts may be offered within religious teachings, spiritual or theological theory or within various kinds of ethical theories. For example, Kant had a theory of virtue, although his moral philosophy would not be characterised (by most people) as a variety of virtue ethics. 'Virtue ethics', on the other hand, bases ethics on virtue evaluation. What we mean by this will become clearer in the course of the chapter, but for now we will follow Swanton's (2003, p. 5) minimal description of what counts as virtue ethics:

> The notion of virtue is central in the sense that conceptions of rightness, conceptions of the good life, conceptions of 'the moral point of view' and the appropriate demandingness of morality, cannot be understood without a conception of the relevant virtues.

The study and advocacy of virtues as excellent character traits has a long and distinguished history within moral philosophy and religious teachings worldwide. The early Chinese philosopher, Confucius (551–479 BCE), for example, wrote extensively about virtue and character, within his broader theory of social duty. For him, the ideal moral character was the gentleman (*chŭn tzu*) whose virtues included benevolence, wisdom and courage (Confucius, 1979 edition). Indeed, within most major spiritual and religious traditions coverage of virtues is prominent – for example, in Islam, Christianity, Buddhism and Hinduism. However, while recognising the richness and diversity of the contributions of a range of cultural and religious traditions to virtue theory and virtue ethics, we have had to be selective. We acknowledge, therefore, that our orientation, inspiration and sources for this book are primarily Western in origin, starting with the ancient Greeks. We also acknowledge that there are many different accounts of the rise, fall and revival of interest in virtues and virtue ethics in Western philosophy, and that the short summary below is just one simplified version.

The early development of virtue ethics

Writing a little later than Confucius, the Greek philosopher, Plato (*c.* 427–347 BCE), put forward the notion of virtue as excellence in the knowledge of the good, which disposes one to the good life and happiness. Plato's list of virtues, developed in several of his dialogues (Hamilton and Cairns, 1961), formed the basis of what became known as the 'cardinal' (basic) virtues: wisdom, courage, justice and temperance. Plato's pupil, Aristotle (384–322 BCE), made what is perhaps the most enduring contribution to a character or virtue-based ethics and his work continues to be discussed and developed today (Aristotle, 1954 edition). Aristotle's ethics emphasises the importance of people aspiring to be good and the connection between virtue and happiness or flourishing. From a Western theological perspective, Saint Augustine (354–420 AD) wrote of the virtuous Christian who obeys the will of God, while Thomas Aquinas (c.1225–1274) brought together Christian doctrine and the teachings of Aristotle. Aquinas added to the four cardinal virtues, proposing the theological virtues of faith, hope and love (charity), which orient humans to the end of union with God (Aquinas, 1993 edition).

Pellegrino (1995, pp. 258–259) characterises this body of thinking as the 'Classical-Medieval' synthesis, rooted in an underlying metaphysical conception (concerned with first principles) of the good of human beings:

> The virtues were traits that habitually disposed humans to act in accord with the ends of human nature – i.e., fulfilment in natural happiness for Socrates, Plato, and Aristotle and supernatural happiness in union with God for Aquinas. On this view, the virtues have normative force not because they are agreeable or admired but because they accord well with, and predispose to, the ends, the purposes, and the good of human beings as defined by an underlying metaphysics.

The decline of virtue ethics

When the possibility of a metaphysical definition of human nature or the good began to be challenged, along with the role of theology, religious authority and reason as a source of morality, then Aristotelian and scholastic philosophy fell into decline. The key role of the virtues in moral philosophy was replaced by a range of alternative concepts, including rights (Locke, 1632–1704), duty (Kant, 1724–1804), moral sentiment (Hume, 1711–1760) and utility (Bentham, 1748–1832). To what extent attention to virtues was marginalised in the works of these philosophers is disputed. Kant and Hume certainly had well-developed theories of virtues (O'Neill, 1996a; Schneewind, 1997). However, although all these theorists had a place for virtues in their ethical theories, it can be argued that virtues were no longer regarded as central.

In the modern period a virtue-based approach became much less popular as the deontological and rationalist approaches of the Enlightenment took hold. MacIntyre (1985, p. 39) describes the Enlightenment project of the period 1630–1850 as entailing the separation of the sphere of the moral from the theological, legal and aesthetic, with the aim of providing a rational justification for morality. The dominant normative ethical theories in modern Western philosophy have tended to be deontological (duty-based, following Kant) and consequentialist (mainly utilitarian, following Bentham and Mill). Other approaches to ethics developed within modern continental philosophy in the nineteenth and twentieth centuries (including existentialism and situation ethics), partly as a reaction against Kant's all-embracing rationalism and separation of ethics from the rest of life. In twentieth-century Anglo-American philosophy there was also a significant trend away from all-embracing universal theories towards linguistic and conceptual analysis (studying the meaning of moral concepts), including developing emotivist accounts of moral judgements (as expressing feelings or preferences, rather than rationally justifiable claims).

The renaissance of virtue ethics

The revival of virtue ethics within recent Anglo-American moral philosophy is usually traced back to a paper by Anscombe (1958). This contained a strong critique of deontological and consequentialist traditions in ethics, which seek a foundation for moral philosophy in notions such as 'obligation' that no longer make sense when there is no law-giver or God assumed. She recommended a move from a focus on obligations to grounding ethics in the notion of virtue, understood as part of human flourishing. Anscombe's article reputedly had a great effect, as some philosophers developed her critique of modern ethical theory while working on developing a virtue-based ethics (Crisp and Slote, 1997a, p. 2).

While it is important to see virtue ethics as a positive development in its own right, the recent revival of virtue ethics has often been framed in terms of a critique of deontological (duty-based) and consequentialist ethics, both of which are based on principles of action (as opposed to the moral qualities or character of the agent). Deontological ethics, particularly associated with Immanuel Kant (1785/1964), the eighteenth-century German philosopher, focuses on principles of right action, with the rightness lying in the nature of the action itself. Consequentialist theories of ethics, of which the best known is utilitarianism, developed by nineteenth-century British philosophers Jeremy Bentham and John Stuart Mill, focus on the consequences of actions, with the rightness of the action being determined by the amount of good produced, often framed in terms of the principle of promoting 'the greatest good of the greatest number of people' (see Mill, 1863/1972). As Statman (1997a, p. 6) comments:

> Principles are just too abstract to provide helpful guidance in the complicated situations met in everyday ethics. These situations typically involve conflicting considerations, to which principle-ethics either offers no solution, or formulates higher order principles of preference, which, again, are too abstract and vague to offer any real help.

Louden (1998) outlines three significant critiques of principle-based theories that have been put forward as arguments to demonstrate their inadequacies when compared with a virtue-based approach. These are briefly summarised as follows:

1. *Principle-based theories offer rule-based models of moral choice.* Reliance on universal principles and rules means these theories tend to be absolutist and ill-equipped to respond to the nuances and particularities of everyday life and practice. Such theories focus on the actions or conduct of the individual rather than on the character of the agent. Virtue ethics focuses on the latter and is arguably better able to accommodate the richness and diversity of the situations in which people find themselves.

2. *Principle-based theories offer rationalistic accounts of moral agency.* Deontological and consequentialist ethical theories tend to focus on rationality and cognition, that is, on how people think and decide with little consideration of the emotions. Emotions and desire are generally thought of in negative terms, as something to be suppressed.

3. *Principle-based theories are excessively formal.* Deontological and consequentialist theories tend to be quite formal, focusing on conceptual analysis and on logical argumentation. They tend also to focus on situations where people have to make difficult

decisions. It might be said that such approaches do not engage with the continuity, narrative or character of the person. They tend to compartmentalise morality or reduce it to specific actions or decisions rather than acknowledge the ongoing and integrated nature of the moral life.

These three types of criticism do not exhaust the accounts of the shortcomings of deontological or consequentialist theories, nor do they render these theories unhelpful. On the contrary, it is useful (particularly to novice professionals) to have guidance from rules or principles. The merits of a virtue-based approach are, it seems to us, most clearly emphasised in relation to the second and third points about rationalism and formalism. While practical reasoning plays a key role in ethical decision-making, this does not preclude a role for emotions or for moral dispositions or character traits. Writing of Aristotle's approach to the virtues, MacIntyre (1985, p. 149) comments,

> Virtues are dispositions not only to act in particular ways, but also to feel in particular ways. To act virtuously is not, as Kant was later to think, to act against inclination; it is to act from inclination formed by the cultivation of the virtues. Moral Education is an 'éducation sentimentale'.

Virtue ethics has now made substantial theoretical headway in mainstream moral philosophy through, for example, the work of Foot (1978), Geach (1977), Hursthouse (1991, 1999), MacIntyre (1985, 1999), Slote (1995, 2001), Swanton (2003) and Williams (1985). Some of these recent versions of virtue ethics are explicitly Aristotelian in origin, others are less so. The amount of literature in this field is growing rapidly, as are debates about particular readings of Aristotle and distinctions between different approaches to virtue ethics (see, for example, Crisp, 1996; Crisp and Slote, 1997b; Statman, 1997b). Much of this recent literature is very much located within the discipline of philosophy and revolves around quite detailed and nuanced debates in philosophical ethics. Arguably the single text with the most wide-ranging impact, not only in moral philosophy, but also in the social sciences and in professional ethics, is MacIntyre's *After Virtue*, first published in 1981 (second edition, 1985). We will offer a more detailed exposition of aspects of this work later in the chapter.

Varieties of virtue ethics

Although there are many varieties of virtue ethics, according to Slote (1997, p. 177; 2000, p. 235; 2001, p. 4), they all share two features in common. First, the main focus is on the individual and those traits, dispositions and motives that qualify him or her as being virtuous. Secondly, in making ethical evaluations, virtue ethics primarily uses terms describing people's character or excellent qualities (such as 'good', 'bad', 'admirable' and 'deplorable'). A definition of virtue ethics suggested by Louden (1998, p. 491) captures most of the key elements:

> Virtue ethics is a theoretical perspective within ethics which holds that judgements about the inner lives of individuals (their traits, motives, dispositions and character), rather than judgements about the rightness or wrongness of external acts and/or consequences of acts, are of the greatest moral importance.

We might question the use of the term 'inner' in this definition as implying (as many versions of virtue ethics do) a distinction between (hidden) inner lives and outer (observable) behaviour. This kind of language is typical of much writing on virtue ethics and will occur in some parts of this book. It should not, however, be taken literally to imply a dualism between internal (motives) and external (acts). The term 'disposition' perhaps usefully captures the holism of 'character in action'.

To reiterate, the primary concern of virtue ethics is with character traits and dispositions rather than action or conduct. The latter are not unimportant, but are explained in terms of virtues. Rather than focusing on the question, characteristic of obligation-based accounts of ethics, 'what should I do?' the question from a virtue ethics perspective is primarily, 'how should I live?' Whereas action-based or obligation-based ethics focus on the rightness or wrongness of actions, virtue ethics takes as its starting point the moral worth of the individual person, which generally (but not always) includes considerations of the nature of the good life and what contributes to it.

Virtue ethics as an all-embracing ethical theory

There are many variations of virtue ethical theory, which differ both in terms of their aims or functions and how they define the virtues and place them in the broader picture of human life. Some versions of virtue ethical theory aim to be *comprehensive, universal and foundational*. By this we mean that they aim to demarcate and cover the whole of the realm of moral life (comprehensive); to apply across all contexts, countries and time periods (universal); and to ground ethics in one core value from which all others can be derived or against which actions or motives can be judged (foundational). A recent example of a philosopher who develops a virtue ethical theory that seems to be making all these claims is Slote (2001, 2007), who draws more on the moral sentimentalism of Hume and Hutcheson than on Aristotle's account of the virtues. He develops a theory based on the foundational virtue of caring, which he argues can do all the explanatory work required to give a comprehensive account of morality, including taking account of justice and giving a general account of right and wrong. Other virtue ethicists might ground morality not in one virtue, but in being a good or virtuous person (someone who demonstrates a range of virtues). This is how Aristotle presented his account of ethics, as do some recent philosophers who have developed a 'neo-Aristotelian' account of virtue ethics such as Hursthouse (1999).

Virtue ethics as complementary or supplementary to other ethical theories

Many theoretical approaches to virtue ethics, however, make more modest claims. For example, instead of developing virtue ethics as a comprehensive account of the whole of morality, resting on one or more virtues or Virtue as a foundational value, virtue ethics might be regarded as one of several theories, which offer *complementary* but incommensurable ways of understanding aspects of the world. We might term this a *pluralist* view, based on the assumption that there are several different, but interwoven and co-existing systems of moral values and moral evaluation, of which virtues and virtue ethics is just one (for a discussion of pluralism in ethics, see Kekes, 1993; Nagel, 1979).

A weaker version of virtue ethics is to see it as a necessary, but *supplementary* part of a broader ethical theory. This approach is more akin to 'virtue theory' rather than virtue ethics, to use the distinction made at the start of this chapter. This approach entails that virtues and theoretical approaches to virtues might be regarded as compatible with and subsumed within an obligation-based or consequentialist theory of ethics. Clearly this is difficult to do without losing the key features of a virtue ethical theory as described by Slote (agent-based with character terms as primary). Kant's (1797/1964) moral philosophy, for example, includes an account of the virtues, but it is presented as part of an obligation-based theory of ethics. As developed by O'Neill (1996b, pp. 185–212), this leads to the idea of obligations or principles of required virtue. Armstrong (2007, pp. 79–82) considers approaches that regard virtue ethics as 'supplementary' to another theory, giving examples from medical and nursing ethics where moral principles and rules are treated as primary, but moral virtues are necessary to provide the motivation for following an obligation or duty (see Beauchamp & Childress, 2001). As Barron (1997, p. 36) points out, in her exposition of Kantian ethics:

> It is a little silly to ask whether a theory is more concerned with action or with character, as if theorists have to favour one over the other. One would expect any reasonably rich ethical theory to be concerned with both, and not to separate them sharply.

Virtue ethics as 'anti-theory'

The accounts of virtue ethics given so far have been in relation to theories of ethics. Many varieties of virtue ethics, however, do not present virtue ethics as a systematic theory or as part of an ethical theory. As Slote (1997, p. 176) points out, there is a tendency for some versions of virtue ethics to be 'anti-theory', based on the argument that the richness and complexities of our understandings of ethical phenomena cannot be captured by generalising theories (see, for example, Baier, 1985; McDowell, 1997; Williams, 1985). If this is the case, Slote suggests, then the study of ethics might be regarded as more like 'history writing or art connoisseurship'. Taking such an approach to the study of ethics might entail giving narrative accounts of our ethical intuitions, based on sensitivity, experience and judgement. Yet while such approaches might not be regarded as 'theories' in the sense of grand, all-embracing theory as described above, they could certainly be described as 'theoretical'. By this we mean that they do involve demarcating the sphere of the 'ethical', and are based on certain presuppositions about what are important areas of study and justifiable ways of accounting for and interpreting matters that fall within the ethical domain.

Virtues based on human flourishing or motivation?

As already noted, all versions of virtue ethical theory have a main focus on the moral qualities of the individual person (as opposed to their actions, or the consequences of their actions). Even accounts of virtues that are supplementary to or framed in terms of another theory, at the point when they deal with virtues, will inevitably have a focus on people's moral qualities or characteristics. Slote (2001) describes this as being 'agent-focussed' – that is, focussing on what philosophers call 'the moral agent', or the person who takes moral action. However, some accounts define virtues in terms of their contribution to human flourishing, and others in relation to the moral agent's motivation.

Neo-Aristotelian accounts of the virtues are often based on human flourishing. Such accounts are termed 'teleological' in that they are based on the idea of an end or 'telos' for human beings, in this case, a conception of the good life in terms of human flourishing. According to Hursthouse (1999, pp. 28–29), who develops a neo-Aristotelian view of virtue ethics, an action is right if and only if it is what a virtuous agent (that is, someone who has and exercises the virtues) would characteristically do in the circumstances. A virtue is a character trait a human being needs to flourish or live well. Hence evaluations of agents and actions are grounded in the concept of human flourishing (a translation of the Greek term 'eudaimonia' used by Aristotle).[1]

Slote (2001), by contrast, explicitly eschews a virtue ethics based on human flourishing, arguing that we derive our ethical evaluation of actions from their relation to people's motives – 'sentiments that reflect a general concern for humanity' (p. viii). These can be

---

[1] According to some critics, this is not, strictly speaking, how Aristotle conceived of the relationship between virtue and flourishing (see Simpson, 1977). Aristotle defined flourishing in terms of the virtues (Aristotle, 1954 edition, 1098a15–b5) rather than grounding virtues in flourishing. His conception of a virtue was actually derived from contemporary Greek culture, which therefore informed his conception of the nature of human flourishing. This points to some issues for eudaimonistic virtue ethics regarding where the notion of flourishing comes from and whether it is grounded in particular cultural and religious traditions, in more specific practices (MacIntyre, 1985), in an intuitive idea of a life worth living or in some revisable and ongoing universal consensus, such as Nussbaum's and Sen's capabilities approach (Nussbaum, 2000, 2006; Sen, 1993).

admirable independent of whether they lead to human flourishing or happiness. He develops a virtue ethics based on the motive of 'caring'. He characterises his view as *'agent-based'*, in that he regards evaluation of moral agents as basic and in no need of justification in terms of human flourishing, as distinct from Hursthouse, who offers merely an *'agent-focused'* view. Slote's account is 'non-teleological' (not directed towards an end) and grounds virtues in intuitive notions of what counts as morally 'admirable' or worthy.

Provided one is not seeking a foundational version of virtue ethics, then it is possible to adopt an approach that includes both teleological (related to an end for human beings) and non-teleological elements. This is what Swanton (2003) does in developing her pluralist virtue ethics. She expresses dissatisfaction with Hursthouse's account based entirely on human flourishing, since this leaves out any considerations of the flourishing of the non-human world, and does not allow for other traits that might be regarded as worthy or admirable, even though they do not contribute to or are not constitutive of human flourishing. Equally, she regards Slote's account of virtues based on motives as too narrow, since she judges that some virtues can be accounted for in terms of their contribution to human flourishing and are regarded as admirable precisely because of this. Swanton, therefore, develops her pluralist approach to virtue ethics, which is not based on any foundationalist claims for justifying or grounding the virtues. Her teleological element takes account of virtues linked to human flourishing, as well as those virtues that do not serve human ends – that is, virtues that serve the flourishing of animals, plants and the non-living natural environment. Her non-teleological element allows for intuitions about virtuousness of traits grounded in their admirability by appealing to the idea of expressiveness. She quotes Hume, who suggests that a 'disutile trait' (that is, one that can not be cashed out in terms of serving any ends), such as 'excessive bravery' or 'resolute inflexibility', can be approved of because of its 'dazzling' qualities or 'ability to seize the heart'. These are virtues not because they serve the end of human flourishing, but because they are expressive of human flourishing (Swanton, 2003, pp. 93–94).

Our version of virtue ethics

There are many other distinctions between types of virtue ethics and numerous debates within the field of philosophical ethics relating to some of the key components of, and concepts relating to, virtue ethics. This includes the nature and role of character, dispositions, motives, emotions, moral luck and blame. This is to be expected, as virtue ethics experiences a revival, then philosophers will get to work to develop, refine, build, demolish and dissect the overall theoretical approach or framework and its component parts. There is a danger of getting so absorbed in this literature that we, the authors, might find ourselves vainly striving to develop our own philosophically sound version of virtue ethics as an all-embracing ethical theory that can then be applied to professional life in health and social care. Yet to do this would not only be a bigger project than we have in mind for this book, it would require us to believe in the value of a standalone, modernist version of all-embracing theory. Whilst, as Hekman (1995, p. 159) points out, moral philosophy is 'one of the last bastions of modernist thought', as practitioner-academics we prefer to engage in a more modest and situated project that explores virtues as one important aspect of ethics in professional life.

Our main aim is to take some of the virtue concepts that seem relevant to professional life in the fields of health and social care and explore them in some detail. This, we believe, is a project that has not been done before, and which takes its starting point from the day-to-day work of health and social care practitioners. So, although we offer an account of some aspects of the history and development of virtue ethics, and some of the key concepts and ideas, we are not attempting to outline virtue ethics as a comprehensive ethical theory covering all aspects of professional ethical life. Rather, we are suggesting that consideration of the moral qualities of individual practitioners is a central part of any study of ethics and any attempt to develop and extend the practice and study of professional ethics. Other features of moral life that need to be considered alongside virtues or moral dispositions include the nature and range of obligations and how we make reasoned judgements and prioritise our duties; what counts as desirable outcomes or consequences of actions and ways of assessing and prioritising these; and the nature of ethical relationships and responsibilities between people and the role of emotions in this. To summarise, we might list the elements of ethics, or sources of moral value, as follows:

- The character of the moral agent (the main focus of virtue ethics);
- The nature of right action (the main focus of deontological ethics);

▶ The outcomes of action (the main focus of consequentialist ethics);
▶ The relationships between people (the main focus of the ethics of care and proximity).

In this book we are focussing on the first element listed above (the character of the moral agent), although all these elements of ethics are intertwined and can be regarded as complementary (addressing different features of moral life). Our view of virtue concepts (such as 'trustworthiness' or 'courage') is that they refer to complex sets of dispositions to feel, think and act in certain ways in certain sorts of situations. A disposition to act in a trustworthy or courageous fashion may be regarded as a virtue (that is, as a morally admirable quality) in so far as it is regarded as constitutive or expressive of human, animal or environmental flourishing. Given that our focus in this book is on professional ethics in health and social care, then our concern in this specific context will tend to be on virtues that are constitutive of human flourishing and could be regarded as grounded (if we regard grounding as important) in the regulative ideals of health and social welfare. The notion of expressive virtues (virtues that express rather than constitute human flourishing, described earlier in connection with Swanton's version of virtue ethics) is not irrelevant to professional life, but is, perhaps, less central.

Thus, to summarise our position in this book: we are offering a theoretical approach or framework (rather than an all-embracing theory); a pluralist view of the sources of moral value (virtues are one important source amongst several); and we regard the contribution to 'human flourishing' as a key element of being virtuous as a health and social care practitioner, while recognising that not all virtues may be of this type.

Virtue ethics and the professions

The revival of virtue ethics in moral philosophy is inevitably influencing the literature in professional ethics, with a small but growing number of monographs developing a specifically virtue-based approach to health care ethics (especially medical ethics), alongside increasing coverage in textbooks where overviews of a range of ethical theories are given, and speculative articles (particularly in social work) suggesting that a virtue ethics approach might be particularly relevant or useful. As Rhodes (1986, p. 42) comments, in her book on social work ethics:

> A virtue-based ethics seems particularly appropriate to professions, because the ethical issues so often focus in the nature of the relationships and our responsibilities in those relationships – to the client, other colleagues, our supervisors, the agency itself. What sort of person ought a 'professional' social worker to be? What is human excellence in that context?

In fact, a focus on virtues, or at least on the moral character or personal qualities of the professional practitioner, was prominent in professional discourse until the latter decades of the twentieth century. Pellegrino (1995) argues that virtue ethics was the dominant normative theory in medicine (and, we might argue, in the professions generally, even if more implicit than explicit) until quite recently. However, it is important to note that the pursuit of medical ethics as a subject of academic study, involving moral philosophical theorising, only really developed from the early 1970s. The systematic study of nursing and social work ethics came even later in the 1980s. So although Pellegrino uses the term 'virtue ethics', he is not literally talking about an ethical theory, nor even a theory of the virtues, rather a focus in practice and in written moral precepts on the good character of the medical professional. He refers to the dominant focus of the longstanding Hippocratic Oath, until recently regarded as the ethical underpinning of medicine, which is partly framed in terms of professional roles and the moral qualities of the practitioner. The updated version of this oath, formulated as the Declaration of Geneva by the World Medical Association in 1948 and revised in 1983 (see Thompson, Melia and Boyd, 2000, p. 340), took the form of a pledge made by practitioners on being admitted as a member of the profession, to practise their profession with conscience and dignity and maintain respect for human life. One of the earliest nursing pledges, formulated by the Farrand Nursing School in Detroit in 1893 and known as the 'Nightingale Pledge', required graduates to:

> Pass my life in purity and to practise my profession faithfully. I will abstain from whatever is deleterious and mischievous and will not take or administer any harmful drug.
>
> (quoted in Thompson, Melia and Boyd, 2000, p. 55)

Here 'in purity' and 'faithfully' can be interpreted as describing the living and practising of the moral qualities of purity and fidelity. Even the later 1960 code of ethics of the National Association of Social Workers in America included a preamble outlining social workers' responsibility to uphold humanitarian ideals and was framed in terms of first person statements, such as: 'I respect the privacy of the people I serve' (Reamer, 1999, p. 44). By the time the British Association formulated a code of ethics (British Association of Social Workers, 1976), the more modern style of principles and rules expressed as action-statements was common, with little or no mention of virtue concepts.

When professional ethics began to develop as a theoretical subject area in medicine, nursing and social work, the dominant focus was on Kantian and utilitarian theories or on middle-range principles combining a focus on duty and outcomes of actions (see, for example, Beauchamp and Childress, 1979; Downie and Telfer, 1980; Veatch, 1981). A notable exception was the work of Pellegrino and Thomasma (1981, 1988, 1993), who developed a grounded theory of the moral relationship between medical professions and the users of their services based on the end or *telos* of the patients' good and from this elaborated a set of virtues. Since then, there has been a growth in attention paid to virtue-based approaches in medical and bioethics (for example, Shelp, 1985; Toon, 1993, 1999), while Oakley and Cocking (2001) offer a well-developed virtue-based account of professional roles in law and medicine.

While some of the writers on medical ethics subsume other health care professions within their accounts, the growth of virtue-based approaches to nursing ethics *per se* is only recently developing, mainly through journal articles and book chapters (for example, de Raeve, 2006; Scott, A, 1995, 1996; Scott, P., 2000, 2003; Sellman, 1997), as well as inclusion in textbooks as one among several alternative moral theories applicable to health care ethics. Sellman's (1997) article is particularly interesting in that it considers and reclaims the virtues (obedience, punctuality and observation) advanced by the nineteenth-century British nurse, Florence Nightingale for contemporary nursing practice. Armstrong's (2007) monograph, while spending a lot of time analysing the inadequacies of obligation-based theories of ethics and summarising the work of MacIntyre (1985), offers what he terms a 'strong, action-guiding' approach to moral decision-making drawing on a neo-Aristotelean virtue ethics.

Interest in virtue ethics is also developing in the field of social work, although more slowly as the study of social work ethics begins to become established. In her book on ethical dilemmas in social work, Rhodes (1986, p. 44) claims to have 'adopted the questions appropriate to a virtue-based ethics'. This involves, she says, considering what our relationships ought to be to our service users, the agency, the profession, colleagues and society; what sort of human excellence we are striving for; and in what social and political context. Whilst Rhodes does give consideration to these questions, she does not explicitly or in any depth develop a virtue-based theory for social work ethics. More recently several articles have appeared advocating the value of a virtue ethics approach in social work (for example, Clark 2006; McBeath and Webb 2002). McBeath and Webb (2002) note that the Greek origins of virtue ethics emphasised relations between public life, morality and individual character, which, they claim, makes it particularly relevant to social work. Textbooks on social work ethics are now beginning to include virtue ethics as one of the available ethical theories (see Banks, 2006; Beckett and Maynard, 2005; Bowles *et al.*, 2006; Charleton, 2007; Hugman, 2005), although hitherto a virtue-based approach has not been fully elaborated for social work.

Human flourishing as a key concept for virtue-based professional ethics

Given the importance of 'flourishing' in virtue ethics, and 'human flourishing' in a virtue-based professional ethics, we will now consider briefly some aspects of this concept. Virtue ethicists who give accounts of human flourishing generally start with Aristotle's concept of 'eudaimonia', of which 'flourishing' is one translation amongst several, all of which have different connotations in English. These include 'happiness', 'fulfilment', 'contentment', 'good fortune' and 'prosperity', and when used as an adjective, 'fortunate, happy, prospering, flourishing, successful, living well' (Hursthouse, 1987, p. 222).

According to Aristotle, living the life of virtue is what constitutes 'eudaimonia', which in turn is the fulfilment of what is the proper function of human beings. Barnes (Aristotle, 1976, pp. 33–34) points out that 'eudaimonia' is not just a mental state but also relates to 'well-living' and 'well-acting'. He says,

The *eudaimon* is the man [*sic*] who makes a success of his life and actions, who realises his aims and ambitions as a man, who fulfils himself.

This suggests that living a good life or flourishing is what human beings aspire towards.

Nagel (1980, pp. 7–14) argues that Aristotle's *Nicomachean Ethics* is indecisive between two accounts of eudaimonia: an *intellectualist account* and a *comprehensive account*. The former is the view that eudaimonia is realised in the activity 'of the most divine part of man [*sic*], functioning in accordance with its proper excellence'. This is the activity of theoretical contemplation. The comprehensive account is where 'eudaimonia essentially involves not just the activity of the theoretical intellect but the full range of human life and action, in accordance with the broader excellences of moral virtue and practical wisdom'. Aristotle's account of eudaimonia is underpinned by what has been called 'the function argument' (see Hughes, 2001, p. 36), which entails that grasping what is the function (*ergon*) of a human being helps us discover what fulfilment or eudaimonia comprises. The intellectualist account focuses on reason and contemplation as the proper function of human beings, which leads to eudaimonia. Alternatively, the comprehensive account allows that eudaimonia comes with participation in a wide range of activities and exercise of the virtues.

In considering the relevance of flourishing to the health and social care professions, the intellectualist account is too narrow. With the exceptions perhaps of professional philosophy and some religious orders, the life of contemplation befits few contemporary professions. The more comprehensive account of flourishing is more attractive, but requires elaboration. How comprehensive need the account of flourishing be in relation to social work, nursing and other health and social care professions?

If we think it helpful to divide virtues into different categories (see Chapter 3), then these can be related to different kinds of flourishing: *moral flourishing* from practising the moral virtues; *psychological or intellectual flourishing* from the intellectual virtues; *social flourishing* from the social virtues; and *physical flourishing* from the physical virtues. *Emotional flourishing* is also relevant and has a more general relationship with the virtues. These categories of flourishing can be related to health and social welfare. They can be compromised by both physical and mental ill-health, by social deprivation and injustice and by the way people are treated within health and social services and in society more generally. Service users' social flourishing may be diminished by physical disability, for example, as they may be subject to discrimination and social exclusion. Their psychological flourishing may also be compromised by symptoms of mental distress such as in dementia and schizophrenia. Service users' physical flourishing may be compromised by physical illness and disability also.

Flourishing is one way of thinking about what we identified in Chapter 1 as the regulative ideals of 'health' and 'social welfare', which could be said to constitute the core social purposes of professionals working in the health and social care fields. Seeing flourishing as relevant in a range of contexts (or categorised into different types) reminds professionals that their actions and omissions may impact on service users' physical, psychological and social flourishing for better or worse. It also enables professionals to think more holistically about themselves. The moral flourishing of professionals is a defensible aspiration in professional ethical development. People are not rational automatons and there needs to be an awareness of the impact of one domain of life on another. An aspiration towards moral flourishing may, for example, compromise physical flourishing as some examples of whistle-blowing demonstrate. Demonstrating moral virtues in the pursuit of the health of others may then damage the physical and mental health of the professional and yet the professional may still have a sense of living well, of flourishing. It needs also to be noted that moral flourishing and other kinds of flourishing are not dependent on each other. Individuals can be healthy, flourish physically and mentally whilst being 'non-virtuous', and can flourish morally and be virtuous whilst unhealthy in other ways.

The good life, flourishing, practices and professions

As already mentioned, for Aristotle the good life is a life lived according to the virtues; and the virtues constitute the flourishing of both their possessor and the wider community. For Hursthouse (1999) and other neo-Aristotelians, a concept of the good life as human flourishing is the starting point of their ethics, and virtues are accounted for in terms of human flourishing. This leads Slote (2001) to comment that these kinds of 'agent-focussed' approaches are less 'pure' forms of virtue ethics, since claims about the good life are explanatorily primary, rather than claims about virtue or moral worth (what is admirable or morally good in people). The concept of 'the good life' may encompass views about human nature, the nature of the relationship between humans, other living and supernatural beings or spirit(s), and what is good for human beings or the planet generally. Not surprisingly, the concept of the 'good life' is generally regarded as highly contested – with many different versions available based on a variety of individual perspectives and cultural, spiritual and religious traditions. It is with this in mind that Enlightenment moral philosophers (mentioned earlier in this chapter) aimed to develop a universal, rationalist theory focused on principles of right action, disentangled (or disembedded) from notions of the good life or individual moral worth that might be located in any particular religious or cultural tradition.

MacIntyre on 'practices'

This is where MacIntyre (1985) starts his account of virtue ethics, bemoaning the fact that although we still have concepts relating to the moral worth of individuals (admirable qualities or 'virtues'), they are not grounded in any conception of the good life, as there are many such contested conceptions. His way forward is to seek to ground virtues within local communities or 'practices'. For MacIntyre, a 'practice' is a complex form of cooperative human activity through which goods are achieved that are internal and external to that practice. External goods could be money, status or prestige. Internal goods are those specific to a practice and include the excellence of the performance and of the product (if something is produced as, for example, an artwork). The achievement of internal goods is also good 'for the whole community who participate in the practice' (1985, p. 190) whereas with external goods there will be competition with winners and losers. MacIntyre gives the games of football and chess and the occupations of farming, painting and music as examples of practices. He does not dwell on professions as practices, but clearly MacIntyre's conception of a practice fits with the concept of a profession as a community of practitioners undertaking activities that are directed towards particular goods and ends. In this context, MacIntyre (1985, p. 191) describes a virtue as:

an acquired human quality the possession and exercise of which tends to enable us to achieve those goods that are internal to practices and the lack of which effectively prevents us from achieving any such goods.

MacIntyre makes a useful distinction between practices and institutions (for example, hospitals, clubs, universities or laboratories). The latter are necessary to sustain practices, but may be more concerned with external goods such as money, power and status. Institutions have the potential to be corrupting and here there is a significant role for the virtues. He writes that:

> The ideals and the creativity of the practice are always vulnerable to the acquisitiveness of the institution, in which the cooperative care for common goods of the practice is always vulnerable to the competitiveness of the institution. In this context the essential function of the virtues is clear. Without them, without justice, courage and truthfulness, practices could not resist the corrupting power of institutions. (p. 194)

Professions as purposive practices

MacIntyre's account of practices is clearly relevant to the professions. Although MacIntyre focuses more on games and occupations such as farming and fishing, he does mention medicine in passing. The idea of the internal goods of a practice could be seen as equivalent to the regulative ideal of a profession that we discussed in Chapter 1. MacIntyre's account of practices has, however, been subject to significant criticism (see, for example, Mason, 1996; Miller, 1994). First, there is the question of whether the notion of a practice based on internally defined and understood good ends or purposes is defensible or helpful. While games, like chess or cricket, can be conceived in this way (with excellence in chess, for example, being recognised and performed in relation to internally generated rules and standards), occupations and professions like farming, nursing and social work have a social purpose. This suggests that their good or end has a reference point outside the practice itself (a comment we made about the concept of a service ideal in Chapter 1). Miller (1994) makes a useful distinction between what he calls 'self-contained' practices like chess and 'purposive' practices like farming. He argues that virtues should be understood as dispositions that sustain *purposive* practices. They are therefore dependent on an understanding of a particular society's dominant purposes and needs.

It is important that there should be an outside reference point for professions as practices. For if we follow MacIntyre's account of practices as more or less self-contained, based on tradition, with no outside reference points against which to judge the internal goods around which the practices are based, this can entail people having to take on very conservative, constraining social roles. This might include, for example, the role of women as carers, or people of minority ethnic origin as slaves. These roles may be functional for the practice, but if they could be judged by an 'outside observer' they might be regarded as oppressive or constraining. If we want to avoid the kind of cultural and moral relativism to which MacIntyre's view might lead, then some concept of the good life (for example, human flourishing, or the flourishing of the natural, living world) that can be accepted as a standard outside particular practices, cultures and religious traditions seems required.

We suggest, therefore, that professions can be regarded as moral communities or practices that have notions of the good or human flourishing built into them in the form of their core purpose or service ideal. This can serve as a reference point for the virtues of the good professional in the context of that profession. So, for example, the good nurse, working to the service ideal of promoting health, might see one of his key roles in relation to a sick person as to be caring. The good lawyer, working to the service ideal of legal justice, might see one of her key roles in defending a case as to be tenacious in pursuing her client's interests. The notion of each profession having a distinctive service or regulative ideal makes sense in these contexts. Yet, as we argued in Chapter 1, and have further argued in relation to MacIntyre's concept of practices, we cannot assume that these service ideals, or core purposes, are independent of the prevailing social and moral norms and values in wider society. The service ideals may be internally agreed and recognised within the professional practices, but they are not divorced from the outside world. For the notion of a profession is based on it being socially sanctioned as beneficial to society. Whilst the ethical norms and values espoused and enacted by professionals within their occupational groups are distinctive from those of everyday life, they are not divorced from prevailing public morality. Rather, as Koehn argues, they should be regarded as an intensification of the ethics of everyday life (the nurse has special responsibilities to be caring or the lawyer to be tenacious, in situations which would not apply in everyday life).

Concluding comments

Virtue ethics is growing in popularity in Anglo-American philosophy and beginning to be applied in the field of professional ethics. Whilst a virtue-based approach has many features that seem particularly appropriate for professional ethics (including its focus on the moral qualities of the professional), we are not convinced that by itself it can provide a complete picture of the whole domain of professional ethics. However, a virtue ethical framework can provide an orientation to professional attitudes and actions that offers a welcome counter-weight to the current emphasis on obligation-based performance to externally defined principles, rules and standards.

We identified concepts derived from the work of MacIntyre (1985), particularly his ideas of complex social practices and shared internal goods, as potentially useful in developing a virtue-based approach in professional life. However, the professions need to be understood more broadly as practices with a social purpose, which ultimately links them to some society-wide notion of the good life, or, more specifically, human flourishing in the domain of health and social welfare.

We have so far only given a sketchy outline of the nature of virtues as complex dispositions involving feelings, thoughts and actions that orient professional practitioners towards the regulative ideals guiding their work, and perhaps ultimately towards some socially recognised conception of human flourishing. In the next chapter the nature of virtues as character traits will be explored further, particularly in the light of critiques of 'character' as a rather simplistic, essentialist notion, which leaves little room for change over time or lapses in ethical conduct.

Chapter 3

Virtues, vices and situations

Introduction

Having outlined several perspectives on the nature of professional ethics and virtue-based ethics in Chapters 1 and 2, we now explore one of the key components of virtue-based ethics, namely the virtues. We consider in more detail what we mean by the term 'virtue' and 'virtues', exploring the nature of the virtues as excellent traits of character. We also examine what is meant by 'character' and 'character traits', considering some of the challenges to the concept of character as comprising relatively stable and enduring dispositions. We will explore different classifications of the types of virtues, the 'doctrine of the mean' and the nature of the 'emotion work' that goes into being virtuous in professional life. The chapter ends by outlining the rationale for our selection of virtues for further study in this book.

Virtue and the virtues

We have already outlined in broad terms what is meant by a virtue-based approach to ethics in professional life and now need to consider in more detail what is meant by the term 'virtue' as used in moral philosophy. One important distinction to make is that between what Adams (2006, p. 32) calls 'capital V' virtue and 'small v' virtue. The former relates to 'persisting excellence in being for the good':

> It ['capital V' Virtue] is the holistic property of having a good moral character. To have it one must not only have a number of

excellent traits. One must have them excellently composed into a whole. When we speak, on the other hand, of particular traits such as benevolence and wisdom, as virtues, we use 'virtue' in a 'small v' sense in which it has a plural and does take the indefinite as well as the definite article.

Labacqz (1985, p. 275) similarly describes virtue as a 'kind of excellence'. She explains that the virtues are 'qualities of character in response to situations', whereas Virtue (if we use Adams' suggested 'capital V' to aid clarity) implies 'an integrity or cohesiveness of character that goes beyond and is different from these individual qualities'.

Our concern in this book is with the virtues, in the plural 'small v' sense. As indicated in the Introduction, it might be more accurate to call our approach 'virtues-based'. However, we have stayed with the common usage 'virtue-based' as this is the terminology used in so much of the literature on the subject.

Virtues as character traits

In describing the nature of the virtues, both Adams and Labacqz make reference to 'character'. Indeed, much of the literature on virtues and virtue ethics describes or defines virtues in this way: as traits or qualities of character. Clearly not all traits of character are regarded as virtues. To be classified as a moral virtue, a character trait must be regarded as morally good or excellent. This is not the only way of describing or defining virtues – sometimes they are spoken of simply as 'moral qualities' or 'moral dispositions'. However, the description of virtues as character traits is such a common feature of virtue-based ethics that it is important to explore the concept of character further and consider some of the critiques of character that have also, by implication, been treated as critiques of virtue-based ethics. Using the terms 'moral qualities' or 'moral dispositions' as alternatives to 'character traits' does not necessarily counter these critiques. Since while avoiding reference to 'character' directly, these concepts are often used in the same way as we use the term 'character traits', to refer to identifiable and persisting dispositions to act in certain sorts of ways. We will now consider, therefore, what is meant by 'character' and 'character traits'.

The nature of character and character traits

In everyday conversation people refer to character in different ways. In relation to a play or film, for example, people might say: 'I didn't think she was a very convincing character'. In relation to someone considered amusing they might say, 'He's a real character'; or referring to someone admired, 'She really has a strong character'. People are also familiar with the idea of giving 'character references' (an account of someone's character in the context of a job application, for example) and may have had reason to ask for or write one for someone else.

The etymology of character is derived (c.1315) from Old French *caractere*, from Latin *character,* from Greek *kharakter* ('engraved mark'), *kharassein* ('to engrave'), *kharax* ('pointed stake'). The meaning, according to the online etymology dictionary (Harper, 2001), is extended by metaphor to 'a defining quality'. Reference to engraving suggests, perhaps, something enduring and brought about by some activity. This is not an uncommon view of character, effectively, as something reliable, stable, robust and, perhaps, relatively unchanging. The idea of character as reliable and stable seems borne out by reflection on our attitudes to those close to us. It does not seem difficult, for example, to provide a character appraisal of friends or family members – describing them, perhaps, as honest, humorous, wise or trustworthy.

Although the terms are often used interchangeably, for our purposes it is important to distinguish between 'personality' and 'character'. According to Goldie (2004, p. 4), a character trait is deeper than a personality trait, and is concerned with someone's moral worth as a person. Personality, on the other hand, is not necessarily connected with moral worth and is often used to describe relatively superficial traits or 'appearances', such as charm, quick-wittedness, introversion, extroversion, gregariousness, shyness or jolliness. Personality describes how a person appears, particularly in social situations. There may be overlap between character and personality; for example, having a warm or friendly personality might also be couched in terms of the virtue or character trait of friendliness. It is possible also for people to be considered as having a good personality (amusing, entertaining, optimistic), but to have a less than exemplary character (perhaps being selfish, ungenerous or dishonest). 'Character' tends to be associated with values and purposes in a way that personality is not. Kupperman (1990, p. 155) puts it this way:

To be committed strongly to moral conduct is not merely to have different goals from some other people or to be different in one's willingness on special occasions to suspend pursuit of ordinary goals. It is to be a different person from what one would have been if one had not been strongly committed. This is linked with a set of values many of which are internal to having a certain character.

These notions of 'commitment' and 'values' are obviously very important in professional life and link with the notion of service or regulative ideals that was discussed in Chapter 1 as orienting professionals towards certain value commitments.

Character is often presented as comprising a set of essential and defining features that is relatively enduring over time and stable and consistent across contexts. There is a sense in which people are considered predictable. If someone is regarded as honest, then there is an assumption or expectation that they are honest across the board, in different ways and in different situations. If someone regarded as honest is involved in dishonest behaviour, then our first response might be to describe this as 'out of character'. However, further reflection on particular cases begins to suggest the complexity of character trait attribution. For example, the notorious London gangland criminals, the Kray brothers, were reputedly kind and loving towards their mother and vicious towards their gangster enemies.[1] Gilligan (1993, p. 104) gives the examples of Martin Luther King and Gandhi, commenting that: 'while the relationship between self and society is achieved in magnificent articulation, both men are compromised in their capacity for intimacy and live at great personal distance from others'. Thus, people who may be considered of exemplary character in some contexts (for example, in political leadership) may be lacking in others (for example, in relation to family). Professionals also have to juggle commitments to those close to them and to their profession. It is eminently plausible that the morally exemplary health or social care professional may be less so in his or her personal life. Indeed, it is questionable whether this tension can ever be truly reconciled as the demands of one sphere may cause the individual to neglect another.

---

[1] We are grateful to Paul Wainwright for suggesting this example.

The situationist critique of character and virtue ethics

Clearly the concept of character and the processes of attributing character traits to people are complex. The examples just given seem to suggest that whether we attribute a character trait to someone (such as being a caring or loving person) may depend upon the context or situation. Some critics of the concept of character, and the way we ordinarily use the term to refer to people's relatively stable and generic dispositions, have pursued this idea of situational variability even further. Many of the critiques offered focus on various psychological experiments that show that it does not seem to make sense to regard people generally as possessing enduring and reliable character traits (such as honesty, courage or cowardice) and to use these to explain their behaviour in particular situations.

In 2007, Zimbardo published *The Lucifer Effect: How good people turn evil*. He describes and reflects on what happened during the Stanford Prison experiment in 1971, when volunteer students were recruited to take on the roles of prison guards and prisoners. The behaviour of the young men who were in the role of prison guards and those in the role of prisoners changed dramatically over the period of the experiment. The former became authoritarian and abusive and the latter powerless and distressed. Zimbardo also discusses other psychology experiments (for example, Milgram's (1974) obedience research) that challenge, significantly, the role of character in explaining such moral lapses. He describes being called as an expert witness to testify for an American prison guard who had worked at the Iraqi Abu Ghraib prison. He discusses the abuse and torture that occurred there and the, seemingly, good character of some of the soldiers. Zimbardo (p. 210) writes of the 'transformation of character' and speaks of, in relation to the prison experiment, 'good people suddenly becoming perpetrators of evil as guards or pathologically passive victims as prisoners in response to situational forces acting on them'. He goes on to say that:

> Good people can be induced, seduced and initiated into behaving in evil ways. They can also be led to act in irrational, stupid, self-destructive, antisocial and mindless ways that challenge our sense of the stability and consistency of individual personality, of character, and of morality. (p. 211)

Zimbardo challenges the 'bad apple in the good barrel' metaphor, arguing that good apples may be corrupted by a bad barrel. The work of Zimbardo and other social psychologists such as Milgram (1974) and Darley and Batson (1973) support the significance of situational factors in explaining ethical failings. The term 'fundamental attribution error' has been used to refer to the mistake people make in ignoring or downplaying factors relating to situations and 'overconfidently assuming that distinctive behaviour or patterns of behaviour are due to an agent's distinctive character traits' (Harman, 1999, p. 315).

This is a potentially challenging critique for a virtue-based approach to ethics in that it may lead to the conclusion that people have no character traits, and hence no virtues, at all. Doris (2002), in a book with the provocative title *Lack of Character*, offers a very full argument in favour of the 'situationist critique', influenced heavily by reports of experiments such as those described above and based on the situationist personality psychology of Ross and Nisbet (1991). Merritt (2000, p. 366) characterises the situationist critique in this way:

> In reality, personal dispositions are highly situation-specific, with the consequences that we are in error to interpret behavioural consistencies in terms of robust traits [...]. Individual behaviour varies with situational variation in ways that familiar concepts of robust traits fail dismally to register.

Our view is that these arguments tend to polarise the discussion of character into either a dispositional or a situational account. Those who focus on situations and ignore individual dispositions might be accused of a situationist error (Merritt, 2000), just as those who focus on individual dispositions and ignore situations might be accused of the attribution error. We would argue that in any given health or social care episode the individual dispositions of the professional and the features of the situation are both relevant to the doing of and the explaining of good actions. This suggests that it is necessary for institutions to support the development of good dispositions or virtues, to compensate for and respond to professional limitations and to aspire to the betterment and non-deterioration of the individual and of the institution, agency or service within which the individual works.

This two-pronged approach is supported by reports from public inquiries that acknowledge individual professional failings, but contextualise these within the organisation and culture. For example, the report of the Bristol Royal Infirmary Inquiry (Kennedy, 2001) into child deaths linked with heart surgery points out that it is not an account of 'bad people', 'people who did not care', nor of 'people who wilfully harmed patients'. The report points to lack of insight and flawed behaviour and discusses deficits in leadership and teamwork and the existence of a 'club culture' where there was an imbalance of power tipped in favour of a few. The Harding Clark report (2006) detailing misconduct at the Lourdes hospital in Drogheda (discussed more fully in Chapter 9) states that 'this is not a simple story of an evil man or a bad doctor' (Harding Clark, 2006, p. 34), and comments that the inquiry team found it difficult to understand why so few people had 'the courage, insight, curiosity and integrity to say: "this is not right" '. The report points to a lack of leadership, peer review, audit and critical capacity. Interestingly neither report suggests that professionals were bad or evil (in what we might call the 'capital V' sense of vice). However, both point to individual failings in terms of lack of insight, courage and integrity (which we might regard as 'small v' virtues) and flawed behaviour, alongside failings in the institutions in terms of lack of leadership and negative cultures.

Clearly there is a complex relationship between the characteristics of people (including their virtues and vices) and the situations in which they live and work. Experiments in social psychology, such as those conducted by Zimbardo and Milgram, suggest that many, but not all, 'normally decent' (Adams, 2006) research participants may be induced to inflict harm on others. Virtues and good character are not, therefore, as robust as we might like to think and there is a dynamic relationship between dispositions and situations. As Adams (2006, p. 158) says,

> We should not be surprised to find that much of what we admire in human beings incorporates a lot of situation-specificity. A person who functions brilliantly in her usual life context may go to pieces in a social situation that is sufficiently diabolical, oppressive, or hostile. But that does not show that the personal qualities that enable her to live so well in the normal range of situations to which she is adapted are not truly excellent.

Any plausible professional ethics needs, therefore, to recognise the potential influence of the situation or context that professionals find themselves in.

To conclude this section, it appears that the situationist critique assumes a version of the concepts of 'character', 'character traits' or 'virtues' that regards these as referring to qualities that are relatively simply defined and are enduring across time and stable between contexts. Clearly we need to conceive of the concepts of character, individual character traits and virtues in a more complex way that allows for situational variation. We will now explore this complexity in relation to our main interest in this chapter, namely virtues.

The complexity of 'virtue' concepts

'A virtue' is often described in singular terms as 'a disposition', 'a character trait' or a 'quality of character'. However, once we stop to think, it is clear that many virtue terms refer to quite complex and heterogeneous clusters of dispositions (attitudinal, motivational and behavioural). Goldie (2000, p. 157), having defined a virtue as a morally desirable or admirable character trait, then goes on to say that:

> character trait terms refer, not to a single disposition, but to a complex network of dispositions which interlock and dynamically interrelate in ways that enable the agent both to recognise and to respond to a situation as embedded in a complex narrative which includes the agent, and his [sic] thoughts, feelings and actions.

This is a useful account of a virtue as it recognises the range of dispositions involved; their interaction with each other and with the specific context or domain in which a virtue is manifested. For example, when someone says of Roshan, a mutual acquaintance: 'Roshan is trustworthy', we take this to mean that Roshan has a tendency to have certain sorts of thoughts and feelings (for example, a commitment not to let people down) and to do certain sorts of actions (for example, to keep promises) in certain sorts of situations (where responsibility and reliability are expected or sought). However, it would be hard to specify more precisely what we might expect of a 'trustworthy' person in a general sense, outside a specific situation or context. Ryle (1949/1973, p. 119) suggests that dispositional statements are law-like in the sense that they license inferences and explanations, but they are also very 'vague'. In the case of 'Roshan is trustworthy', we might infer from this statement that Roshan is not routinely going to lie to people, but we cannot make specific predictions about Roshan's motivations and actions in particular contexts.

Adams (2006, p. 125ff) suggests that it might be useful to regard virtues as 'modular' – that is, as consisting of more or less independent component parts from which a complex structure can be assembled. He gives the example of honesty, suggesting that we tend to group under the one heading 'honesty' a variety of different traits that are commended by different reasons or have different roles. So a person may be honest in one sense or context, but not in another. For example, a young person may never lie to a close friend, but will cheat in examinations. Adams suggests that some modules of a virtue may be regarded as 'domain specific', that is, relating to attitudes and/or behaviour manifested in certain types of situations – such as with friends or in examinations – or in specific social roles. As a social role, he gives the example of being a parent or a stockbroker. Given our interests in this book, we could add, being a nurse or a social worker.

Several writers make similar points when analysing individual virtues, using slightly different terminology. For example, in discussing integrity, Mussshenga (2001) distinguishes 'global integrity' which applies across all roles and domains of life, from local integrity (in a particular role or context). Potter (2002) distinguishes what she calls 'specific trustworthiness' from 'full trustworthiness'. Specific trustworthiness refers to trust that is specific to certain relationships, while full trustworthiness is a disposition to be trustworthy towards everyone. According to Potter, it is the latter that is a virtue. This suggests she regards a virtue as a relatively enduring and stable character trait. This would entail that people we term 'trustworthy' would behave in a trustworthy fashion across all contexts. If they failed to behave in a trustworthy fashion on a particular occasion or in a specific context (for example, if they broke a confidence), then we might expect an explanation, justification or excuse (for example, someone's life was in danger; they had a lapse of memory). If this was not forthcoming or satisfactory, then we might say that either they are not trustworthy (in the full sense) or they are trustworthy in some contexts and not in others.

In Chapter 7 on trustworthiness, we use a vignette featuring a social worker, Alison, who is regarded by Helena, the woman she has worked with for several years, as trustworthy. Alison is reliable, she is committed to supporting Helena and she keeps her promises as a social worker. This is the only context in which Helena knows Alison. However, let us assume that in her leisure time, Alison plays tennis with a friend, Margaret. As a tennis partner, Alison's behaviour is quite unreliable. She often comes late to the tennis club and sometimes even misses games she has arranged with Margaret. She promises to improve her game and practise her serves, but never finds time to do this. She has repeatedly said she will come on time and do more practice. But this never happens. Margaret decides not to choose Alison as her partner in a tennis tournament because she says Alison is not trustworthy.

What should we say about Alison's trustworthiness? We could take several different approaches to this. First, assuming 'trustworthiness' to mean global or full trustworthiness, and if we do not take account of any possible explanations or excuses, then we might say, 'Alison is not trustworthy'. By this we might mean either that she lacks the global virtue of trustworthiness or, perhaps, that she has the vice of untrustworthiness. A second possibility, still taking 'trustworthy' to refer to global trustworthiness, but taking account of extenuating circumstances, might be to say,

Alison is basically trustworthy, but she has problems with her elderly mother who keeps calling her in the evening. Alison feels she has to respond, hence missing her tennis practice and being late for her games. She knows this is not a good way to behave towards her tennis partner, but finds it difficult to manage her time and her relationship with her mother at present.

This suggests a basic trustworthiness, with an excuse/justification offered for Alison's lapses in the context of her tennis commitments. Finally, if we consider the concept of trustworthiness as modular, and look at Alison's local or situation-specific behaviour, then we might say, 'Alison is trustworthy as a social worker, but not as a tennis partner'. Alison will hold to her promises and be reliable in work-related matters when vulnerable people rely on her, but tends to be late or miss appointments in personal life.

Although we often talk about virtues in the first global sense, as if it made sense to characterise someone as completely and utterly trustworthy across all situations and roles, in fact, this is a very difficult interpretation to put into practice. Our characterisation of someone as trustworthy is based on the context in which we know them. So although we make what appears to be a global claim when we say 'Alison is trustworthy', it is based on local evidence, and is, to some extent, context or situation dependent. If we are not to be surprised or disappointed at people's attitudes and behaviour, then we do need to bear in mind the situated nature of people's dispositions. Indeed, while 'folk psychology' leads us to talk in terms of character traits being stable and enduring, we do have well-recognised means of accounting for 'out of character' behaviour, in terms of mitigating circumstances or excuses, for example, as Goldie (2000, pp. 167–175) points out. The complexity and modularity of the concept of 'character' itself and of particular character trait concepts (such as 'trustworthiness' or 'courageousness') means that we might not be particularly surprised if someone is regarded as trustworthy or courageous in one context but not in another. Although we find it useful to talk in terms of character traits and virtues, these are not fixed and simple dispositions. We will now move on to consider virtue theorists' classifications of virtues, which relate to the types of contexts and situations in which they are deployed.

Types of virtues

Many theorists distinguish different kinds or types of virtues. Some of these distinctions are useful in helping us understand the nature of the rather heterogenous collection of concepts characterised as virtues. However, the categorisations often used may tie that particular virtue concept to a rather narrow field of operation. Given that we have suggested that virtues are complex and modular, then categorising them in relation to a specific domain of operation tends to imply a more simplistic account of virtue concepts than that to which we would subscribe. We will give an account of some of the different ways in which virtues have been categorised, but the reader should bear in mind that some of the distinctions made assume a rather essentialist, simple and reified (the idea that virtues actually exist as objects) view of the concept of a virtue.

Distinctions are often made between different general types of virtues, based on, or developed from, some of the classifications of Aristotle. These include distinctions between moral, intellectual, physical and social virtues; between genuine and simulacra virtues; between self-regarding and other-regarding virtues. There is even a recent concept of 'burdened' virtues, although this is a much more situational account of how a particular moral quality (such as care or courage) can be a burden to its 'possessor' in certain contexts (for example, in situations or relationships that are oppressive).

With the exception of professional wisdom, the virtues discussed in this book could be classified as moral virtues – care, respectfulness, trustworthiness, courage, integrity and justice. This makes sense regardless of whether we think we are classifying the virtue in itself or the domain in which it operates. However, once we start to think about these categories they may not be particularly helpful. Justice is also often categorised as a 'civic' virtue, and courage can be categorised as 'moral' in some contexts and 'physical' in others. Professional wisdom is generally regarded as an intellectual virtue. The intellectual virtues are outlined in book VI of Aristotle's *Nicomachean Ethics* as: episteme (science or scientific knowledge); *techne* (art or technical skill); *phronesis* (prudence or practical wisdom) and *nous* (intelligence or intuition). Aristotle outlines the physical virtues in *The Art of Rhetoric* (1991 edition, p. 87) as 'health, beauty, strength, size and competitive prowess'. The relationship between social virtues (such as politeness, sociability and wit) and moral virtues is interesting in relation to virtues such as respectfulness. It may be that social virtues can have a moral dimension contributing to the flourishing of individuals but they may also be superficial: *simulacra virtues* rather than *genuine virtues*, a matter of performance rather than being for the good. There may be disagreement as to what is a 'genuine' and what is a 'simulacra' virtue. The virtue of agreeableness, for example, was considered by Aristotle to be a simulacra virtue, while Jane Austen considered it a genuine virtue, in fact, a prerequisite for other virtues (MacIntyre, 1985, p. 183).

A distinction is also often made between *self-regarding* and *other-regarding virtues*. There is generally held to be an asymmetry in duty-based ethics between ethics in relation to ourselves and ethics in relation to others (Statman, 1997a, p. 5). On an obligation-based approach to ethics people are, and it is held should be, more concerned with the interests and well-being of others than with their own interests. This is not the case with virtue ethics, where one's own flourishing is as significant as that of others. Taylor and Wolfram (1968, pp. 238–248) set out the distinction as follows:

> a man [*sic*] possessing the other-regarding virtues will benefit others, while a man possessing the self-regarding virtues will benefit largely himself.

Temperance, prudence, courage, circumspection and industry are given as examples of self-regarding virtues. Generosity, conscientiousness, compassion, kindness, honesty, veracity and justice are described as other-regarding virtues (Slote, 1997, p. 192; Taylor and Wolfram, 1968, p. 238). It does not seem to us that these categories are mutually exclusive. The moral virtues, discussed in this text, are both self-regarding and other-regarding. Courage, for example, has the potential to contribute to the professional's flourishing in that it enables him or her to overcome fears and achieve ends. Service users benefit as the courageous social worker or nurse will be able to support them at difficult times and bear their fear, anger and loss. Courage is also a factor in enabling a professional to speak out against poor practice. Respectfulness takes two forms: self-regarding (self-respectfulness) and other-regarding (respectfulness). Again both are necessary for professional practice. The virtues of care, trustworthiness and integrity also appear to have both dimensions.

Slote (1997, p. 196) specifies a useful principle in relation to the self-/other-regarding distinction, as follows:

> One should be concerned to promote one's own well-being and virtues and also concerned to promote the well-being and virtues of other people.

This is an approach we support as necessary within a virtue-based professional ethics. However, we accept that it is not always the case that the promotion of one's own well-being is compatible with the promotion of virtue, that is, with flourishing in general. While the well-being of a nurse or doctor may be promoted by cutting short a painful consultation with a service user, this may not be compatible with the virtues of care or respectfulness. There is also evidence to support the view that the exercise of some virtues (courage in relation to whistle-blowing, for example) is detrimental to the physical or psychological well-being of professionals, although it is possible that their moral flourishing will be enhanced. Tessman (2001, 2005) introduces the concept of *burdened virtues* to describe the virtues that people living under conditions of oppression may be required to develop and which carry a moral cost for those who practice them. In her analysis of political resistance, for example, she argues that the excessive demand for courage takes its toll on its bearer:

> The courageous disposition that the political resister is encouraged to cultivate and to foreground in his/her character may crowd out other virtues in a deleterious way.
>
> (Tessman, 2005, p. 125)

Virtues commonly regarded as 'feminine', such as caring, can promote self-sacrificial traits, meaning that women may be disproportionately involved in promoting the flourishing of others at the expense of some aspects of their own flourishing (Okin, 1994). A quotation from Rafferty (1996, p. 40) relating to nursing in the nineteenth century suggests this, with the nurse expected to be: 'firm yet gentle in her manner, eager to learn and devoted to her work', with a manner that conveys 'the impression that it is in the sickroom where she finds her appointed field of sacrifice'. Clearly this turn of phrase does not encapsulate the virtues that would be required in twenty-first century nurses, although the tendency still remains for the virtue of caring to take on an element of self-sacrifice. If caring is taken to excess, however, it may transform into an attitude of martyrdom, and we would probably tend to regard this quality as a vice rather than a virtue. This leads us to another topic in the literature on virtues that it is important to consider, namely, their relationship to vices, and the work that people have to do to achieve 'being virtuous'.

Virtues, vices and the doctrine of the mean

On Aristotle's account, the right expression in relation to the virtues or dispositions has been described as 'the doctrine of the mean'. This is the idea that virtues and vices come in triads with each virtue flanked by two vices (vicious dispositions) – one representing excess and one deficiency (Barnes in Aristotle, 1976, p. 26). In relation to courage, for example, the doctrine of the mean points to the vices of excess (foolhardiness) and of deficiency (cowardice). The mean is not necessarily a mid-point. Aristotle (1976, 1106a20–b9) gives the example of food for an athlete. The trainer's knowledge that two pounds of food is too little and that 10 pounds is too much will not lead the trainer to conclude necessarily that six pounds is the mean and the correct amount as this may still be too much or too little. The circumstances will determine the mean not the centre point on an excess/deficiency scale.

The doctrine of the mean is a useful way of thinking about the ethical dimensions of professional practice as it encourages professionals to consider the emotions that emerge in professional practice and the right expression of them. The idea that dispositions are in a mean and need to be expressed in the right way, towards the right object and in the right amount is however a challenging idea. So too is identifying the relevant feeling or emotion in relation to each virtue and specifying what would appear as excess or deficiency. Carr (1991, pp. 55–56) identifies problems with what would count as excess honesty and justice, for example. He also states that:

> the doctrine of the mean is the perfectly reasonable idea that the passions and appetites are not as some philosophers have suggested merely sources of temptation to be controlled by the virtues, but actually necessary conditions for the expression of them. By this I mean not only that courage would not be possible without fear but also that charity and compassion would not be possible in the absence of genuine human feelings of love and concern for other people.

In relation to the virtues discussed in this book, in Table 3.1 we attempt to identify how excess and deficiency would appear in relation to each virtue. The exercise also enables us to consider what might be considered vices in relation to each virtue. This task is more challenging in relation to some virtues than others. For example, in relation to courage, an excess characterised as foolhardiness and a deficiency as cowardice seem well accepted. For virtues such as trustworthiness and integrity it is more difficult to find single vices that would be regarded as an excess or deficiency of those qualities. This is not surprising, given our account of the complexity of virtue concepts. Indeed, several commentators question the usefulness of the doctrine of the mean. Slote (1997, p. 184) suggests that while it might work for the virtues of courage and justice, it is not appropriate for many of

Table 3.1 **Professional virtues and vices**

Vice – Deficiency	Virtue – Mean	Vice – Excess
Indifference or callousness	Care	Excessive/smothering concern
Disrespectfulness	Respectfulness	Extreme deference Servility
Excessive partiality	Justice	Extreme indifference
Extreme unreliability	Trustworthiness	Punctiliousness
Cowardice	Courage	Foolhardiness
Superficiality	Integrity	Inflexibility

the virtues emphasised in modern moral philosophy, such as honesty and truthfulness. Truthfulness, for example, is not about telling neither too much nor too little of the truth. Slote's point is an important one, and is a useful reminder not to take the 'doctrine of the mean' too literally. Its usefulness is more, perhaps, in that it indicates the amount of work (emotional, cognitive and sometimes physical) that a moral agent has to do in order to develop the virtues and act in accordance with them.

Emotions, 'emotion work' and the virtues

We will now explore further this idea of the work that the moral agent has to put in to being virtuous, in particular what has been called 'emotion work'. One of the areas of criticism of principle-based ethical theories discussed in Chapter 2 is that they are overly rationalistic, too focused on cognition and rationality, with scant regard for the role of the emotions in the moral life. One of the positive features of virtue ethics is that, rather than advocating a suppression of the emotions, it accommodates their appropriate expression. In order to develop this feature of virtue ethics further, we need to consider the nature of the emotions, which emotions are relevant and how they relate to the moral life more generally and to virtues more specifically.

The emotions (*pathos*) and feelings (*pathé*) are central to Aristotle's ethics. Aristotle's virtue ethics entails the right expression or moderation of the passions or emotions 'in the right place and at the right time' (Carr, 1991, p. 50). In the *Nicomachean Ethics*, Aristotle describes virtues as dispositions and relates this to feelings or emotions (for example, desire, friendliness, anger, fear, daring, envy, joy, jealousy, pity, hatred, longing). He explains,

> By disposition I mean conditions in virtue of which we are well or ill disposed in respect of the feelings concerned. We have, for instance, a bad disposition towards anger if our tendency is too strong or too weak, and a good one if our tendency is moderate. Similarly with other feelings.
>
> (Aristotle, 1976, 1105b2–26)

It can be said that a virtue-based approach is a matter of feeling well in addition to acting well. As Kosman (1999, p. 264) puts it: 'the art of proper living [...] includes the art of feeling well as the correlative discipline to the art of acting well'. The use of the term 'emotion' by many of the recent philosophers concerned to rehabilitate the role of emotion in ethics (see, for example, Blum, 1994; Goldie, 2000; Nussbaum, 2001; Oakley, 1992; Vetlesen, 1994) is generally based on an understanding of 'emotion' as having a cognitive element. Vetlesen (1994, p. 78) argues that 'in a distinct emotion there is a blend of affectivity and cognition'. He distinguishes this from a feeling, which is 'rawer' and has a quality of being so close that the subject is virtually engrossed in it. Emotion, on the other hand, involves a step back, and 'adds an element of reflection absent in the feeling', signifying a more mature stance towards the object of emotion and a stronger element of interpretation and evaluation. This echoes Blum's (1994, pp. 173–182) account of the 'altruistic emotions' (such as empathy, sympathy and compassion, which are grounded in a concern for the 'weal and woe' of others), which can be distinguished from 'personal feelings' (such as liking and affection, which are grounded in personal, but not necessarily moral, characteristics of the other person). Hursthouse (1999, p. 118) suggests how ethical responsiveness is dependent on emotions and also discusses the limitations of rules without emotional engagement:

> the whole idea that a human agent *could* do what she should, in every particular instance, while her emotions are way out of line, is a complete fantasy. Our understanding of what will hurt, offend, damage, undermine, distress or reassure, help succour, support, or please our fellow human beings is as much emotional as it is theoretical [...]
>
> the grasp of, and adherence to, the rules would *still* not take us all the way to 'what we should do'. For sometimes 'what we should do' is just, as we say, 'be there' for other people. They tell us what they have suffered, and the tears come to our eyes; they tell us what they have endured and our faces flush with indignation or anger. It is all in the past, there is nothing we can do to undo it, no comfort or assuagement we can offer in the form of action. Such comfort and assuagement as we can offer, as we should, springs solely from our emotional reactions. If we can't come up with the right ones, we fail them, and it is a moral failure.

Although we would challenge Hursthouse's view that comfort and assuagement in such situations stem solely from emotional reactions, we agree that appropriate ethical responses need to be informed by reason *and* emotions. The emotions, so often ignored or downplayed in professional ethics play at least three roles, which we will outline briefly.

1. *Emotions contribute to motivation* – we feel moved to act when we experience certain emotions. Stocker (1976) discusses the devaluation of the emotions in some modern ethical theories. He argues that 'the person' is missing from utilitarian and deontological approaches and there is a disconnection (a 'schizophrenia') between reason and motive. People can act rightly towards others but their action lacks 'moral merit or value' if it is not motivated by appropriate emotions such as friendship, love, affection, community and fellow-feeling. These emotions are an important part of moral motivation. Without fear, anger, love and concern we would be less likely to act in ethically appropriate ways.

2. *Emotions also enable us to respond sensitively* to people's suffering and anguish, as Hursthouse describes in the extract just quoted. They counter the potentially dehumanising effects of principle-based ethics.

3. *Emotions prompt us to appraise ourselves or others* when, for example, we experience moral emotions. Emotions can help distinguish ethical from unethical behaviour. For example, a professional might feel disgust when confronted by racist or ageist attitudes and discriminatory behaviour. She may feel shame or guilt if she fails to live up to her service or regulative ideal. Stempsey (2004, p. 50) describes shame and guilt as 'emotions of self-assessment' providing a means of self-evaluation and comparison, of how things are with how they could or ought to be. The emotions provide visceral signs that all is or is not well ethically and can be described as embodied responses. A more general emotional reaction is that of moral distress, whereby people experience negative emotions as a result of not being able to do what they believe to be the right thing or doing the wrong thing (McCarthy and Deady, 2007). In everyday practice, professionals may feel fear, anger and sadness. Emotions are evoked and experienced in practice situations – a professional may feel frightened when confronted by an aggressive relative, angry when a service user is denied a service considered helpful and sad when someone dies.

These three points suggest that moral agents have to do a considerable amount of work in the sphere of feelings and emotions in order to develop and practise the moral dispositions or virtues. Health and social care professionals often work in very challenging circumstances. They may find it difficult to demonstrate care towards those with whom they work to enable them to feel cared for or they may not always have the feelings or emotions they think appropriate towards service users or others. They may, effectively, lack the relevant emotional response and virtuous dispositions. The concept of 'emotional labour' is useful in helping us understand how professional practitioners can handle such situations. This is a phenomenon identified by the American sociologist, Hochschild (1983), in her study of Californian students, flight attendants and bill collectors. She defined emotional labour as: 'the induction or suppression of feeling in order to sustain an outward appearance that produces in others a sense of being cared for in a convivial safe place' (Hochschild, 1983, p. 7).

Emotional labour involves two kinds of emotion work: surface and deep acting. The former involves our consciously changing our outer expression 'in order to make our inner feelings correspond to how we appear'. Deep acting involves our changing our feelings from the inside so that the feelings 'we want to feel show on our face' (Smith, 1992, p. 7). Deep acting requires that people work on their feelings, generating a 'real feeling that has been self-induced' (Hochschild, 1983, p. 35).

The concept of emotional labour has been explored in relation to nursing (see Smith, 1992; Smith and Gray, 2001) and can also be applied to other caring professions. Smith's emphasis is a little different to that of Hochschild, as she describes emotional labour or work as intervening 'to shape our actions when there is a gap between what we actually feel and what we think we should feel' (Smith, 1992, p. 7). James (1989) researched emotional labour in the context of a hospice:

> The management of emotions has many of the connotations associated with labour as productive work but also the sense of labour as difficult, requiring effort and sometimes pain. It demands that the labourer gives something of themselves and not just a formulaic response.
>
> (cited by Smith, 1992, p. 6)

At first sight it might appear that emotional labour is anathema to a virtue-based approach, as it suggests acting and, perhaps, performing what Aristotle described as 'simulacra' rather than 'genuine' virtues. However, what seems central to emotional labour is the realisation that the management of the emotions of the worker or professional is crucially important in his or her ability to provide care and a sense of safety. Furthermore, it is acknowledged that professionals are not always able to feel appropriately on cue, to demonstrate the appropriate virtue always and everywhere. Emotional labour is compatible with a view of professionals as social actors playing a role with nothing implied about their motivational dispositions. It is also compatible with a virtue-based approach whereby the wise professional recognises that this labour is necessary for the expression of the virtues. Emotional labour is particularly relevant to moral virtues with a relational focus, for example, care, trustworthiness and respectfulness. It is also, arguably, part of the process of habituation necessary for the expression and development of the virtues. Necessary conditions for emotional labour compatible with a virtue account would seem to include the ability to reflect on one's practice and to ask how this emotional labour relates to the narrative of one's overall character and to the *telos or ideal* of one's profession.

Which virtues?

A large number of virtues are relevant to the caring professions. Some lists of virtues have been proposed by philosophers and others by ethicists with a particular interest in the professions. These have been summarised in the table in the Appendix at the end of the book. At least some of the so-called 'cardinal' or basic virtues (courage, justice, temperance and prudence/practical wisdom) are evident on most lists and the theological virtues (faith, hope and love/charity) evident on several. Our selection of virtues for this text is based on what we believe a well-rounded picture of the professional life requires, but is not designed to be exhaustive. The rationale for courage, professional wisdom, respectfulness, trustworthiness, care, justice and integrity over some other virtues is, therefore, based on three main factors:

1. Professionals need to perceive well, deliberate appropriately on the conduct and character of themselves and others and make

decisions within specific social contexts. They need to respond to limitations in rationality, sympathy and resources and to express moral virtues appropriately. *Professional wisdom* enables practitioners to do this and can be considered as a virtue relevant in contexts where recognition of the salient features of situations, moral imagination, deliberation and decision-making are required.

2. Evidence from social sciences supports the view that professionals are vulnerable to corruption in certain social and institutional contexts and need to have virtues that render them more resilient and capable of resistance. Virtues such as *courage, integrity* and *justice* might, as suggested by MacIntyre (1985), be required to resist institutional corruption. These virtues might be thought of in some circumstances as virtues relevant to this kind of resistance.

3. One of the primary goals of health and social care professionals is to contribute the promotion of human flourishing and to do this they need to be able to develop meaningful relationships and to respond appropriately to human vulnerability, distress and achievement. Virtues such as *care, trustworthiness* and *respectfulness* might be thought of in these contexts as relational or responsive virtues.

The virtues we have selected are necessary but not sufficient for the caring professions. We allow, for example, that a wide range of other moral and non-moral virtues may well enhance health and social care practice, for example, humility, honesty (in relation to self-scrutiny, for example) and humour. Indeed, a variety of different virtues has been suggested for the medical, health and social work fields, a few examples of which are given in the Appendix at the end of the book. However, we feel that our choice of virtues for further study is wide-ranging enough to cover rather different types of moral virtue and small enough to allow an in-depth discussion of each chosen virtue.

Concluding comments

In this chapter, as part of the process of elaborating on the nature of virtues, we questioned the concept of character and character traits as referring to easily identified properties of an individual that can be specified outside the particular contexts in which they are manifested. Although we often do tend to attribute good character and good or admirable character traits in this way as part of our everyday ways of talking and understanding, these concepts are much more complex and situation-dependent than our ordinary language suggests. We suggested that virtues, as excellent character traits, need to be understood as complex dispositions, which may be modular in nature.

Professionals might be described as of excellent or exemplary character if they demonstrate composite virtues in all domains. It seems to us, however, that it is somewhat utopian and idealistic to insist that all professionals demonstrate all of the relevant composite virtues all of the time. Good character does require, however, that they display most of the modules of the relevant virtues in the professional domain most of the time. As Adams (2006, p. 201) suggests,

> It is wise to assume that we are all 'mixed bags', good and bad in different respects, and that differences in moral performance reflect differences of situation as well as of character.

The chapters that follow begin with accounts of aspects of real-life practice depicted in vignettes that have been composed to illustrate some of the complexity underpinning any understanding of virtues in relation to everyday health and social care practice. Some of these vignettes are drawn from the literature, and others from interviews conducted for this book, or other research projects, as outlined in the Introduction to the book.

Chapter 4

Professional wisdom

Introduction[1]

Health and social care professionals make judgements and act on decisions in complex and often uncertain circumstances. Guidance in practice protocols and codes is likely to fall short in prescribing what exactly should be done and how. Rules, protocols and prescriptions cannot cover every eventuality and there will be exceptions to these. Professionals may, for example, be uncertain regarding the requirements of honesty in certain situations. Respect for confidentiality is not an absolute obligation and there will be circumstances when sharing information without service user consent will be necessary. Professionals provide care to service users but it may not be appropriate that they should always intervene in anticipation of some future harm. Such examples suggest that technical expertise and rules are insufficient. They suggest also the need for perception and deliberation in relation to the particularities of practice situations. Practice situations are rarely resolvable solely by technical or clinical expertise. In the face of complexity and uncertainty, 'professional artistry' is required in addition to technical competence. Such artistry encompasses ethical responses that are not simply formulaic or rule-bound, but are related to the personal and moral qualities and dispositions of the practitioner, in particular, the virtue of practical wisdom.

---

[1] Some of the material in this chapter draws on an unpublished PhD thesis (Gallagher 2003).

In the ancient Greek literature on the virtues, *phronesis*, often translated as 'practical wisdom' or 'prudence', is categorised as one of the four cardinal or basic virtues (the others being courage, justice and temperance). As noted in Chapter 3, *phronesis* is regarded as an intellectual virtue, and is often considered a precondition for the moral virtues. It is a virtue required for ethical decision-making and action and for the development of the moral virtues. In this chapter we will use the term 'practical wisdom' to refer to the generic virtue of *phronesis*. After examining the nature of practical wisdom, we will then focus our attention on 'professional wisdom', that is, practical wisdom in a professional context. This includes the ability of professionals to perceive the salient features of particular situations; to deliberate well; to make decisions and to act in ways that contribute to the appropriate demonstration of the virtues and the flourishing of those involved in professional life.

Vignettes

The examples in this chapter come from interviews with a senior physiotherapist, Joe, and from Samina, a drugs worker in a voluntary sector (not for profit) organisation. Joe shares his view of professional wisdom and reflects on an example from his own practice. Samina discusses how she tries to promote equality in her practice and shares some concerns regarding appropriate responses to service users.

1) Misdiagnosis: a view from physiotherapy

Joe describes people he believes have demonstrated wisdom in their professional work.

> I've certainly met physiotherapists who have wisdom. I often think of it as the art of therapy – people who – the textbook assessment would say you start at A and you get to Z – they skip and they move from A to P to wherever. And they also know what works and what doesn't work without actually having to go through that situation. And you just get this, sort of, nice feeling from those people. I think of examples of wisdom – I can think about my team manager at the moment actually, it's not a practical example but we sit and we have team meetings and discussions every couple of weeks regarding clinical issues. She will sit there and someone will describe everything that's going on with a client and then she'll ask, like, the

most pertinent question that nobody has even thought to ask. You know, like she's got thirty years of experience as a physio[therapist] working in the community. She knows, she's got this, like, inherent understanding of what the issues are. I think it's difficult to have wisdom without having understanding. She knows what the issues are for clients in our community and she can ask those questions.

Joe outlines a situation that he was involved in. A junior physio-therapist had been visiting a woman at home for some time, providing physiotherapy two or three times a week. The woman had been complaining of knee pain and did not seem to be improving. Eventually the junior therapist asked Joe to visit with her.

I went in and had a look. Not to blow my own trumpet, it sounds a bit bad, but when I went in to have a look I said: 'this is not a knee problem, this is a hip problem and actually I think this is quite a serious hip problem'. So we came back to our consultants, who are attached to our team, and said: 'Can you have a look at this lady?' They reviewed the notes. They said: 'Look, she's been in hospital, she's been into A and E [Accident and Emergency] twice with this issue, she's had her knee x-rayed, she's had her hip x-rayed, there's not a problem'. Maybe it's a sign of courage, I basically had to say: 'This woman has a hip problem and she's potentially got a broken hip and we need to look at this and we need to do this properly'. And it turned out that she did, she actually had a fractured hip. So, you know, did I have wisdom or not? You know, she'd been to A and E twice, she'd been x-rayed but just going in there, taking a look at her in the bed, having a chat and sort of, looking at how she said she'd done it. And luckily or unluckily she actually ended up spending about three months in intensive care, she spent another two months lying on flat bed-rest and, sort of, had a horrendous history in the meantime. But I think I was quite proud at that moment. I felt that my experience, my wisdom about, about how people would normally present allowed me to be able to go in there and say: 'You know, none of the rest of this other stuff matters; what we need to get done right at this point is this'. So I suppose it's maybe seeing the wood for the trees sometimes.
(Source: interview)

2) Recognising needs and advocating for a service user

In an interview with Samina, a drugs worker, she was asked what she thought the core values were that she operated within as a drugs worker. She mentioned promoting equality and challenging inequality. She also added,

> I suppose it's to be as open and honest as much as I can be [...] just to kind of work in a way that's equal to everyone and also to be, kind of, true to myself, not to just go in there and be one person when I'm at work and another person when I'm at home sort of thing.

Samina shared her concern about the approach of other workers:

> Some staff have had a homeless client, they've taken their washing home and done their washing. Some staff have brought in clothes or shoes, whatever, that they might have had left over from their children. I don't know of anybody that's actually gone out and bought something for a client, although the team leader did buy one client lunch on her birthday which caused upset because she hadn't bought any of the other clients lunch on their birthdays [...] But people are kind of mothering the clients in a way and that doesn't sit quite right with me but then again you feel awful because you might have something spare that somebody needs.

She described her own approach to a client who needed a cooking stove. Instead of giving him one, she gave him a leaflet with information as to how he could get a cheap stove for himself. Samina provided a rationale for her position as follows:

> I would rather look at what the situation is and how they can change it and where they can go, because there are charities that will give out tents and stuff like this, so that's more the way I would go rather than crossing the kind of boundary I've got with the client. I'd point them in the direction of other people that can help, but other things they can do themselves that sort certain things out. I think we'd get too messy if we just became people that snapped our fingers and everything was sorted because that doesn't teach them anything,

they don't learn anything, they don't move forward at all. So [...] I don't want to operate in a benevolent way because it is quite clear that we do make more money than they make because most of them aren't working and we do have a lifestyle that's completely different from theirs. And if we come in with all these things that they need it just emphasises the gap between the workers and the clients.
(Source: interview)

Reflections

The perspectives of Joe and Samina suggest interesting dimensions of wisdom and expertise in everyday practice. Joe describes wise physiotherapists he has known in terms of their ability to move beyond the textbook assessment. Their ability to 'skip and move from A to P' rather than working from A through to Z suggests flexibility and responsiveness to the particularities of situations. He talks also of the 'art of therapy' and of the wise physiotherapist 'knowing what works and what doesn't work'. Regarding the wisdom of his manager Joe refers to her asking 'the most pertinent question that nobody has even thought to ask' and of the importance of understanding and of knowing what the issues are for these particular clients.

The example Joe discusses regarding his own work with a more junior therapist relates to an initial misdiagnosis. The service user had been treated, unsuccessfully, for a knee problem when she actually had a hip problem. In relating this to wisdom, Joe talks of how he listened to and looked at the woman. He uses the metaphor of 'seeing the wood for the trees'. The ability to discern, to perceive well, to listen, to see and to draw on previous experience seem relevant to Joe's description. His discussion suggests technical judgement and skill. Although things may not have worked out so well for the service user who 'had a horrendous history in the meantime', his intention was, it seems, to diagnose correctly and to alleviate her discomfort. Joe's description of the work of physiotherapists who, he believes, have wisdom suggests also tacit knowledge and the ability to be flexible and not rule-bound. Whether Joe's intervention represents professional wisdom will be considered below.

Samina discusses the importance of being open and honest and of being true to herself. She shares her concern and uncertainty about the approach of some of the other workers, for example, in doing service users' washing and giving them clothes and shoes. She gives the example of a staff member buying a birthday lunch for one service user and not others and suggests that this caused upset. Samina talks of other workers 'mothering' service users, but acknowledges that sometimes 'you feel awful' because you may be in a position to give. Her response to a service user who needed a cooker was to give him a leaflet so he could get a cheap cooker for himself. Interestingly, Samina is critical of what she describes as operating 'in a benevolent way' and prefers to 'look at what the situation is and how they [service users] can change it'. Her stance then suggests the promotion of independence and, perhaps empowerment, helping service users to 'move forward'. Samina suggests that, for her, giving to service users merely emphasises the gap, or perhaps, inequality, between workers and service users. Samina does not discuss wisdom but her reflection on her everyday practice suggests that she is sensitive to the ethical dimensions of practice and, more particularly, to the expression of virtues such as openness and honesty.

Practical wisdom – background

Practical wisdom is an intellectual virtue if we follow Aristotle's categorisation. The intellectual virtues are outlined in Book VI of Aristotle's *Nicomachean Ethics* as: episteme (science or scientific knowledge); *techne* (art or technical skill); *phronesis* (prudence or practical wisdom); and *nous* (intelligence or intuition). A distinction is also made between *phronesis* and *sophia*. Whereas the former is generally associated with practical wisdom, which relates to decision making in particular situations to achieve a good, the latter relates to theoretical wisdom, concerned with the contemplation of the nature of things in a universal sense. However, caution needs to be exercised as *sophia* is sometimes used to mean practical wisdom (Devettere, 2002). There are different philosophical perspectives on practical wisdom in ancient philosophy (for example, from Aristotle, Socrates, Plato and the Stoics). Here, we focus on the perspective of Aristotle and describe professional wisdom as *phronesis* or practical wisdom as applied to a professional context.

Practical wisdom appears as a virtue in many of the world's philosophical and religious traditions (Humphreys, 2005). For the Chinese philosopher, Confucius, wisdom is a virtue concerned with applying knowledge well. Buddhist 'nirvana' is described as a 'fusion of virtue and wisdom – the latter operating in this particular context as a moderating or harmonising influence on the human character' (Humphreys, 2005, p. 157). Hinduism similarly emphasises the relationship between being good and being wise. Stories of the 'wisdom of Solomon' appear in Jewish, Christian and Islamic literature (Humphreys, 2005).

Aristotle assumes a central role for practical wisdom as an intellectual virtue that governs or enables the right expression of the moral virtues. Comte-Sponville (2002, p. 32), using the term 'prudence', puts it this way:

> Prudence [practical wisdom] does not reign over the other virtues (justice and love each have more merit); it governs them. And indeed, what would a kingdom be without government? Merely loving justice does not make us just, nor does loving peace make us peaceable by itself: deliberation, decision, and action are also required. Prudence determines which of them are apt, as courage provides for their being carried out.

Within the somewhat reified version of the virtues offered by Aristotelian theory, we could say that without practical wisdom the other virtues would be rudderless. The examples in the introduction and in the narratives from Joe and Samina suggest the complexity, subtleties, uncertainty and different professional perspectives within everyday practice. Even when it is clear what virtues are indicated – for example, when people feel frightened they might recognise the need for courage – it is not always clear whether this is a situation that warrants courage nor how much courage and towards what end. Courage alone cannot tell us what actions are appropriate. We use the term 'practical wisdom' to encapsulate people's perceptual and deliberative capabilities to respond ethically.

Features of practical wisdom

Devettere (2002) offers a detailed account of *phronesis*, which he translates as 'prudence'. Although he uses the term 'prudence', we will continue to use 'practical wisdom' except when making direct quotations. Devettere suggests that five features of practical wisdom can be identified from observing how virtuous people live: that practical wisdom is acquired deliberately; that it is *the* decision-making virtue; that it involves reasoning about what is good and bad; that it relies on experience; and it provides ethical norms for action. Each of these features has relevance to professional wisdom.

What is meant by practical wisdom being required deliberately, the first feature identified by Devettere (2002, p. 112), is that it is 'a state of mind acquired thoughtfully and deliberately for its own sake'. That is, the practically wise person becomes wise by doing wise things. This is a thoughtful, intentional and deliberate process rather than a mindless habitual one. Habit results in people doing things repeatedly without reflecting on them: for example, putting three spoonfuls of sugar into their coffee, having a cigarette after dinner or clearing the table between courses. These habits are not virtues and do not require reflection. Like the other virtues, practical wisdom requires a reflective habituation. The more people reflect and are conscious of what contributes to the development of practical wisdom, the wiser they are likely to become.

In describing practical wisdom (prudence) as *the* decision-making virtue, the relevance of the virtue to professionals becomes clear. Devettere (2002, p. 112), drawing on Aristotle, distinguishes amongst three phases of decision-making:

▶ Deliberation (*bouleusis*) – This involves working out what action in a particular situation will contribute to 'doing well and living well' or to flourishing. The deliberation relates to areas where choices are to be made and where people have to decide whether one thing rather than another is good for them to do. People may choose to consult with others if the decision is a major one.

▶ The decision itself (*prohairesis*) – A distinction is made between choice, which does not require deliberation, and a decision which follows from deliberation. Animals and young children can make choices but not decisions;

▶ The command (*epitaktike*) that leads to action – This requires that people go beyond deliberation. Practical wisdom, therefore, commands people to do what they have deliberated on and decided.

Practical wisdom, then, involves deliberation, decision-making, commands (or prescriptions) and the execution of a decision. Devettere (2002, p. 113) distinguishes between making prudential decisions and making moral judgements. The latter are not, he says, decisions as they do not require personal actions. People might, for example, debate and draw conclusions about the ethics of euthanasia or abortion, but they are not engaged in a prudential decision if they are not deciding about something they will actually do. Although practical wisdom is described as an intellectual virtue, it is a very practical one as it leads to action in the real world. Such action is directed towards the good. The wise or prudent person is one who 'implicitly knows what is good for human beings – what would conduce to their fulfilment and thus eudaimonia – and who acts intelligently in accord with that understanding' (van Hooft, 2006b, p. 67). People learn how to become wise also by observing people who are wise, observing how they manage their lives and live well.

Practical wisdom involves reasoning about what is good and bad. This is the third feature suggested by Devettere (2002, p. 115). He describes it as a 'truth-attaining reasoning'. Prudential reasoning is different to the reasoning that may be used in science. Prudential reasoning involves working out what to do in particular situations to achieve something good. It is always directed towards something that is 'truly good'. This good is human flourishing. Such reasoning relates to the expression of the virtues in everyday practice.

Practical wisdom also relies on experience. Devettere (2002, pp. 116–117), again drawing on Aristotle, discusses the importance of experience in moral decision-making. He points out that practical wisdom (prudence) is

> above all concerned with particulars – a particular person in a particular situation is making a particular decision about a particular action in an effort to achieve a particular life that will be good and bring personal happiness – and understanding particularity comes from experience […]. Prudence is based on the personal experience of actually living a moral life. Its truth is practical because it is based on human experience, not on theories about how we ought to live. The theoretical knowledge found in moral theories is not capable of resolving the problems that people encounter in trying to live well […] The virtuous person, not the moral philosopher, is the better guide for ethical action.

Devetterre points out that although young people may be proficient in mathematics and science they lack the experience needed for wise or prudent decision-making. These comments also highlight an interesting feature of a virtue-based approach, that is, what is required to live well cannot be derived from theory. To become virtuous we need to look to people considered virtuous rather than moral philosophers. People who have an impeccable grasp of the nuances of ethical theory may not, of course, live an ethical life.

Although there is no algorithm that will resolve the dilemmas of professional practice, decision-making frameworks have been devised that prioritise and provide guidance on key values in different areas of life (business, education, health and social care). Ethical codes also provide ethical guidance in the form of duties or obligations. Ethical theory does not offer a panacea for all moral ills but it does provide language and guidance that enables people to engage in discussion and to appreciate what values are relevant and what is acceptable and not acceptable in specific situations. As discussed in Chapter 2, it is not our view that it is only virtue ethics that provides insights into the moral life. However, it is clear that understanding individual virtues and discerning what is required in specific situations does require practical wisdom.

The fifth and final feature of practical wisdom discussed by Devettere (2002, p. 117) is that it is the 'norm for moral action'. People live by their own right or prudential reason rather than by the dictates of moral laws, rules or principles. Where the person is virtuous he or she will choose to live a good life, will reason rightly, desire appropriately and consequently flourish and may contribute to the flourishing of others. However, what of those (most of us) who are less than virtuous? Devettere argues that, whereas those who are virtuous have no need for laws, principles or rules, the latter do have a role in helping people to be good and to avoid bad actions. People who act in accord with rules, duties, obligations or laws have some way to go before they can be said to deliberate, decide and act in accord with practical wisdom. Such repeated actions may, however, over time lead to the development of practical wisdom and other virtues.

The features of practical wisdom (and, by association, professional wisdom) outlined by Devettere are helpful in deciding what might be considered prudential or wise. In relation to the examples of Joe and Samina it is difficult to draw firm conclusions about their wisdom. It seems possible that, as with the other virtues, they might have demonstrated some but not all modules of professional wisdom. Joe is able to cite the example of a more experienced colleague he considers wise suggesting he might learn from her example. He then reflects on a clinical example that shows him using his professional experience and expertise to give a new diagnosis of a patient's problem. Joe can be seen as deliberating and deciding and this resulted in action. Joe's use of the metaphor of 'seeing the wood for the trees' and his ability to draw on previous experience suggests technical expertise, perhaps, rather than moral virtue. It is unclear whether Joe aspired to the overall flourishing of the service user and himself or if his focus was on physical flourishing. He does not talk explicitly about the virtues but his actions might suggest some of the professional virtues discussed in this book, for example, courage and trustworthiness.

Samina refers more explicitly to virtues, referring to openness and honesty. She discusses a particular instance of giving an advertisement to a service user directing him to where he might buy a cooker he needed. Samina's account shows her reflecting on, perhaps agonising about, the ethics of her practice. She does consider the ends of her practice, although not in relation to the broad ideals of health and social welfare. She discusses them rather in relation to moving service users on and helping them to become more independent and, perhaps, empowered. She is concerned about equality in connection with relationships between service users and also service user–worker relationships. Samina's ability to deliberate and to act on her decisions and also her reflection on the ends of her practice, on relationships and on the expression of virtues suggest that she is practically or professionally wise in some ways. Given that the information in the vignettes is limited and we do not have access to the larger biographical narratives of both professionals, it is not possible to say with any certainty whether they are wise people or not, but it does seem plausible that they aspire to the flourishing of the service users with whom they work. It may well be that only a virtuous person working closely with Joe and Samina in their practice contexts over a long period would be able to determine whether they demonstrate practical wisdom or not. We turn next to the nature of professional practice.

Everyday practice and professional wisdom

Professional practice has been characterised in different ways. Schön (1987, p. 3), for example, describes the 'swampy lowland' of professional practice where 'messy, confusing problems defy technical solution'. Uncertainty, ambiguity and complexity are features of the 'swampy lowland' of everyday professional practice. Schön goes on to say that professionals crave the 'high, hard ground' where problems are amenable to technical solutions. However, it is in the swampy lowland that professionals will most often find themselves and it is here that professional expertise is manifested.

Fish and Coles (1998) have characterised practice in a similar way. They distinguish between the *technical rational* (TR) view and the *professional artistry* (PA) view of practice. Fish and Coles (1998, pp. 31–33) write of the TR view as follows:

It views professional practice as a basic matter of delivering a service to clients through a pre-determined set of clear-cut routines and behaviours. The metaphor of 'delivery' has become so common that it appears as an unquestioned part of discussion in both health care and education [...]. The TR view then, characterises professional activities as essentially able to be pre-specified and susceptible to being broken down into their component parts [...] Such skills, it is assumed, can be listed beforehand, and are commonly referred to as competencies, or, sometimes, 'performance outcomes' [...] The technical rational view of professionalism and the competency approach to practice is rapidly gaining ground as the only view.

Fish and Coles (1998) critique this view of professional practice, arguing that it makes incorrect assumptions about the reliance on guidance and protocols and about professional judgement. The TR approach does not acknowledge the significance of professional judgement nor does it enable professionals to develop and refine this. Schön also emphasises the importance of problem setting. People do not approach professionals with simple technical problems that can be fixed by a simple TR solution; their problems are complex and the role of professional expertise is to understand what the problem really is and how best to help the person.

The alternative view is the PA view which challenges the TR view, arguing that practice cannot be simplified and made predictable as the TR view suggests, but rather should be approached as complex and uncertain (in keeping with Schön's 'swampy lowland'). Fish and Coles (1998, p. 35) write:

The professional artistry approach sees professional practice as complex. Just as a painting, a poem or a piece of music demands a response to its entirety which would not be satisfied only by analysing it technically into its component parts, so professional practice needs to be understood holistically.

Table 4.1 **Technical rational and professional artistry views
(adapted from Fish and Coles, 1998, p. 41)**

The technical rational (TR) view	The professional artistry (PA) view
Emphasises:	Emphasises:
▶ Rules, laws, protocols and prescriptions	▶ Patterns and frameworks
▶ Diagnosis and analysis	▶ Interpretation and appreciation
▶ Efficiency	▶ Creativity
▶ Knowledge as graspable and permanent	▶ Knowledge as temporary and dynamic
▶ Theory as applied to practice	▶ Theory emerging from practice
▶ Evidence and what is known	▶ Uncertainty and ambiguity
▶ Assessment, appraisal and accreditation	▶ Investigation and reflection
▶ Training	▶ Education
▶ Technical competence	▶ Professional judgement

A summary of the two views of professional practice is presented in Table 4.1 (adapted from Fish and Coles 1998, p. 41).

There is a role for both the TR and the PA views in responding to the complexities and uncertainties of health and social care practices. A much more integrated view is necessary. It seems possible, therefore, to distinguish between practical wisdom and technical or clinical expertise. Illustrations of judgement and decision-making in relation to both views are evident in the vignettes. Joe, for example, talks of assessment guidance running from A to Z (TR view) and of the need for professional responses that are more flexible, acknowledging the particularity of individual situations (PA view). A TR view is evident in his response to a technical problem of mistaken diagnosis and inappropriate treatment. Samina appears to have to rely more on professional judgement and artistry (PA view) as there does not appear to be a clear TR response. To be proficient in professional artistry requires more than rote learning and pre-determined behaviours. It requires professional wisdom, that is, practical wisdom in professional life. Discussion of clinical judgement that distinguishes between technical and humane judgement (Downie and MacNaughton, 2000) supports the distinction between judgement that has to do, primarily, with technical or clinical matters and that which has to do with the development of relationships and the moral dimension of practice.

Professional wisdom

The features of practical wisdom (prudence) discussed by Devettere in the last section are relevant to the professions and to professional wisdom. Most crucially, in relation to the caring professions, professional wisdom requires perceptual and reflective elements. In writing of these elements in relation to the work of a lawyer, Kronman (1987) writes of wisdom joining reflective and perceptual elements together as a 'synthesis'. He also writes of the significance of the imagination.

Professional wisdom is the wisdom necessary for professional practice, requiring, we suggest, the following elements:

▶ an understanding of the role of TR and PA views of professional practice as discussed earlier;
▶ an ability to perceive the ethical dimensions of practice and to appreciate what is salient;
▶ the exercise of the moral imagination;
▶ reflective and deliberative capabilities to make decisions and to act.

There is overlap between the exercise of perceptual and reflective capabilities and the moral imagination and it may seem that these capabilities are exercised simultaneously. We have already discussed the TR and PA views. We now turn to the other dimensions of professional wisdom.

An ability to perceive the ethical dimensions of practice and to appreciate what is salient

In discussing difficult cases with student professionals they may say, 'I didn't see that as an ethical issue'. The students may, for example, be discussing a technical or procedural issue (for example, resuscitation or safeguarding children procedures). They may, therefore, perceive some aspects of the situation – the technical or clinical dimension – but not the most salient from an ethical point of view. People may, therefore, recognise some aspects of the situation but not others. They may not see something as an issue at all, moral or non-moral. They may not have a finely tuned sense of moral perception.

Blum (1994) gives the example of Joan and John who are travelling on a full underground train. A woman is standing holding two shopping bags. Joan is aware that the woman is uncomfortable, whereas John has not noticed this. Their awareness of the situation is different or, as Blum puts it, exists 'at different levels' (1994, p. 32). Their view as to what is more or less salient is different. Blum puts it this way:

> In this situation, the difference between what is salient for John and Joan is of moral significance. Joan saliently perceives [...] the standing woman's good (i.e. her comfort) as at stake in the way John does not. Joan perceives a morally relevant value in the situation that John does not.

What is morally significant in the situation, according to Blum, is the relationship between perception and action: 'John's perception provides him with no reason to offer help to the woman' (pp. 32–33). Blum comments that John's perceptual failing in this situation suggests

> a defect in his character – not a very serious defect, but a defect nonetheless [...] John's failure to act stems from his failure to see (with the appropriate salience), not from callousness about other people's discomfort. His deficiency is a situational self-absorption or attentional laziness. So there is a different moral significance to failing to act depending on the character or explanation of that failure (pp. 33–34).

Blum's suggestion that John is deficient by being self-absorbed and lazy in his lack of attention to the woman's plight is challenging. This can be related to the phenomenon of 'moral blindness', discussed by Johnstone (2004) where people do not see the moral dimensions of situations. Johnstone (2004, p. 92) likens this to colour-blindness: 'just as a colour-blind person fails to distinguish certain colours in the world, a morally blind person fails to distinguish certain "moral properties" in the world'. As with many of the moral qualities discussed in this text (such as good character or courage), it is not the case that people either have them or lack them, but rather that they may demonstrate degrees or modules of the quality or capability and this may also vary according to the circumstances. For example, John may tend to be poor at noticing people's discomfort on the subway, but very highly tuned to the comfort of his clients when making a business transaction. Alternatively, on another occasion, when he is less self-absorbed, John may be highly alert and notice other people's discomfort on the subway.

Blum's position that failure to see the morally salient features of a situation results in inaction is persuasive: if people, professionals or non-professionals, do not recognise the moral features of a situation, for example, a person in need or a social injustice, then they are unlikely to respond ethically. However, there appear to be good reasons why people do not, and should not be expected to, respond to every person in need or every social injustice. First, people are likely to be overwhelmed by the enormity of need and social injustice. Second, their resources are limited and they would be unable to meet every need or fight every social injustice. Third, they are likely to become less able to engage with personal, social and professional commitments due to their preoccupation with responding to the ethical dimensions of every situation perceived. If, for example, a social care worker is escorting a service user on a shopping trip they would, appropriately, focus on the needs of this particular service user, rather than be engaged in scanning the scene with a view to spotting signs of discomfort, need or injustice in other people generally. There are, therefore, good reasons why apparently limited moral vision should not always be viewed as suggesting character defects, and factors can be suggested in mitigation. John might, for example, have been preoccupied with another ethical issue or situation (perhaps worrying about Joan's health or concerned about the well-being of an older person on the other side of the carriage). 'Moral blindness' (or 'moral blind spots') may, as Blum suggests, be influenced by and contribute to character deficits. If, for example, a person's racism, sexism, homophobia or ageism result in their not perceiving or ignoring the morally salient features of a situation, then this might mean we attribute character shortcomings to that person.

How this discussion relates to the health and social care professions can be illustrated by returning to the vignettes. Joe describes the wisdom of his team manager who listens and then asks 'the most pertinent question that nobody had even thought to ask'. This suggests that perception is not only related to the observation of behaviour but also to picking up verbal cues, the salient features of a description or discussion, responding appropriately, providing guidance and modelling a professional response to those less experienced. In discussing the example of his visit to see the woman who had been misdiagnosed, Joe talks of 'taking a look at her in the bed, having a chat and sort of, looking at how she said she'd done it'.

He uses a visual metaphor explicitly towards the end of his account when he says, 'I suppose it's maybe seeing the wood for the trees sometimes'. Joe's discussion of professional wisdom focuses on examples where practitioners had listened and observed, identified salient features and then responded. The examples suggest professional artistry and are ethical in nature as they concern the flourishing of the service user and others. Joe does not discuss the role and response of his more junior colleague when Joe provided an alternative diagnosis. Might this also have been a salient feature of the situation? The flourishing of colleagues can be enabled or thwarted in such situations. Samina appears to perceive at least some of the salient features of her work situation and demonstrates sensitivity to the predicament of service users. She considers also how it might be for service users to receive second-hand goods from workers stating that this reinforces a 'gap'. Such thoughts suggest that Samina is considering the perspectives of others. At times, this requires the exercise of the moral imagination.

Moral imagination to expand the scope of concern

There are situations in personal and professional life when it is particularly difficult to care, to be respectful, courageous or kind and to 'be for the good'. Such situations might involve not liking or understanding a person in social life or at work, perhaps a colleague, student, service user or carer. The person may be positively disliked, disapproved of or perhaps even disgust us for any number of reasons. Perhaps the person is racist, sexist or homophobic or perhaps they express behaviours that are intimidating or insulting. There are few situations when exercising the moral imagination will not provide another perspective enabling us to look again and to learn of other dimensions of the person concerned.

The philosopher, Iris Murdoch (1970) gives the example of a woman, M, who does not like her daughter-in-law, D. M's initial evaluation of D is, for the most part, negative. She perceives D to be unpolished, lacking in dignity and somewhat immature. Over time, M reconsiders her view of D and decides to 'look' again. She concludes that rather than being vulgar D is 'refreshingly simple', rather than D being noisy she is bright and cheerful, rather than immature D is 'delightfully youthful'. Murdoch, also using the metaphor of vision, writes of M seeing in a particular way:

What M is *ex hypothesi* attempting to do is not just to see D accurately but to see her justly or lovingly [...] M is engaged in an endless task.

(Murdoch, 1970, pp. 22–23)

And,

I can only choose within the world I see, in the moral sense of 'see' which implies that clear vision is a result of moral imagination and moral effort [...] The moral life on this view, is something that goes on continually, not something that is switched off in between the occurrence of explicit moral choices.

(Murdoch 1970, p. 36)

Murdoch's 'seeing' or 'looking' requires effort and can indicate moral progress or regress. Emotional labour, as discussed in Chapter 3, is also a component of this effort. Professionals in health and social care sometimes work with service users they find difficult. Liaschenko's (1994) work provides examples. She points to the importance of attentiveness and of looking for 'the commonalities of need' we all share. It seems that, in situations where professionals find service users challenging, there is much opportunity for ethical betterment or progress. Such progress can be enabled by practising the just and, perhaps, loving or respectful looking suggested by Murdoch.

Rather than seeing a service user as, for example, attention-seeking and demanding, the exercise of imagination can lead to a reinterpretation of the situation – what is really going on with this service user? Perhaps her anxiety-provoking or challenging activities are the only way he or she can assure staff attention. It is suggested that 'seeing' the situation in more ethical terms can alter professional actions. It requires, however, the ability to engage in self-scrutiny and to allow oneself to be challenged by and to challenge colleagues and others. Engaging the imagination is, it seems to us, a component of the deliberation engaged in as part of professional wisdom.

Reflective and deliberative capabilities to make decisions and to act

One of the features of practical wisdom referred to by Devettere (2002), and discussed earlier, is decision-making. Devettere's (2002, p. 112) three phases are deliberation; the decision itself; and the command leading to action. Aristotle's kind of deliberation is represented by what is called a 'practical syllogism' – a set of premises that lead to a conclusion. Hughes (2001, p. 94) gives the following example:

1. Physicians aim at producing healthy patients.

2. Removing Annabel's appendix would restore her to health (the hidden premise being that 'Annabel's appendix is inflamed – she has appendicitis').

3. So, I should have Annabel's appendix removed.

Hughes points out that there is evidence of 'particulars' and 'universals' in this example. 'Particulars' relate to what is particular or special about, and what should be done, in this individual case. 'Universals' relate to a more generalisable level of deliberation which includes views of the role of physician, patient diagnosis and an understanding of health. Professionals need professional wisdom to decide what should be done in this case or particular situation, here and now; and to maintain a focus on the overall nature and the regulative ideals of the professions. Deliberation or reflection involves thinking, requires knowledge, the ability to scrutinise oneself and the circumstances one finds oneself in, the ability to make judgements and to act on those judgements. It is both a philosophical and a practical activity.

In relation to philosophy, Blackburn (1999, p. 5) distinguishes between 'knowing how' and 'knowing that'. He points out that thinking skills or engaging in reflection is not just about the acquisition of a body of knowledge – it is a 'knowing how' as much as a 'knowing that'. He points to the example of Socrates who

did not pride himself on how much he knew. On the contrary, he prided himself on being the only one who knew how little he knew (reflection, again). What he was good at – supposedly, for estimates of his success differ – was exposing the weaknesses of other people's claims to know. To process thoughts well is a matter of being able to avoid confusion, detect ambiguities, keep things in mind one at a time, make reliable arguments, become aware of alternatives, and so on.

(Blackburn, 1999, p. 5)

This resonates with the vignettes described earlier. The interventions of Joe and Samina suggest a 'knowing how' as well as a 'knowing that'. They also suggest the importance of honesty and humility in relation to one's own professional knowledge and skills.

Schön's (1983) book, *The Reflective Practitioner: How Professionals Think in Action*, initiated a significant development in the professions embracing reflection as a legitimate educational strategy. Schön identified a dichotomy between the 'hard' knowledge of science and scholarship and the 'soft' knowledge of artistry and unvarnished opinion. This resonates with the discussion of technical rationality and professional artistry above. Professional 'knowing', according to Schön, begins with the assumption that competent practitioners usually know more than they can say. He discusses the 'crisis of confidence' in the professions and points to the 'tangled web' and complexity of healthcare practice. There is now a very large and growing literature relating to reflection and the professions and there continues to be debate as to what reflection really means (see, for example, Rolfe *et al.*, 2001; White *et al.*, 2006).

While there are many definitions of reflection, the following features tend to be regarded as important: contemplation with a view to uncovering knowledge; a change of conceptual perspective: and a process that involves action. For reflection to be meaningful in relation to ethics it has to relate to action. Two types of reflection are further highlighted: reflection on action and reflection in action. Reflection on action involves 'the retrospective analysis and interpretation of practice in order to uncover the knowledge used and the accompanying feelings within a particular situation' (Atkins and Murphy, 1994, p. 51). Reflection in action involves recognising and thinking about a new situation while acting. Reflection in action is an important component of ethical practice. Professional wisdom requires both reflection in action and reflection on action. The ability to reflect on oneself, on one's own ethical conduct and character is fundamentally important. MacIntyre (1999, p. 71) writes of the importance of reflection in relation to moral development:

> What each of us has to do, in order to develop our powers as independent reasoners, and so to flourish qua members of our species, is to make the transition from accepting what we are taught by those earliest teachers to making our own independent judgements about goods, judgements that we are able to justify

rationally to ourselves and to others as furnishing us with good reasons for acting in this way rather than that.

In addition to the ability to stand back from and to be able to evaluate our desires, to engage effectively in self-scrutiny, MacIntyre (1999, p. 96) also points to the possibility of fallibility regarding self-reflection and highlights the importance of social relationships in affirming and correcting self-knowledge. He writes:

> We may at any point go astray in our practical reasoning because of intellectual error: perhaps we happen to be insufficiently well-informed about the particulars of our situation; or we may have gone beyond the evidence in a way that has misled us; or we have relied too heavily on some unsubstantiated generalization. But we may also go astray because of moral error: we have been over-influenced by our dislike of someone; we have projected on to a situation some phantasy in whose grip we are; we are insufficiently sensitive to someone else's suffering. And our intellectual errors are often, although not always, rooted in our moral errors. From both types of mistake the best protections are friendship and collegiality.

MacIntyre (1999, p. 97) gives good reasons for the importance of friendship and collegiality but also points to the possibility of fallibility whereby friends and colleagues may lack the virtues necessary to develop and sustain practical reasoning.

Professional wisdom is a virtue that guides professional practice so that professionals perceive the salient features of practice situations, exercise their moral imaginations, appreciate the need for scientific and humane judgement and, crucially, make ethical decisions. Professional wisdom equips professionals to demonstrate the appropriate moral virtues in the right way in relation to practice situations.

Strategies for practice and professional education

Engaging with the humanities, particularly literature

Incorporating the humanities, particularly literature, into professional programmes has been suggested as a means to develop the perceptual or seeing capabilities of professionals. Attention to stories or narratives in practice (for example, the stories of Joe and Samina) or fiction may develop student professionals' ability to appreciate better the patient or service user's perspective and to enhance their abilities in moral perception. This is also suggested by Montgomery Hunter *et al.* (1995):

> More specifically, literature has been included in the medical curriculum to develop students' narrative competencies, for example, the capacity to adopt others' perspectives, to follow the narrative thread of complex and chaotic stories, to tolerate ambiguity, and to recognise the multiple, often contradictory, meanings of events that befall human beings.

The humanities or arts, particularly literature, can then bring students closer to and make them better able to appreciate the patient and professional experience. Students may also learn to exercise their moral imagination, in the way discussed by Murdoch, and to be able to formulate more humane and respectful hypotheses about an individual's experience or behaviour which may, initially, appear inexplicable and chaotic. Nussbaum (1990, p. 95) also reminds us that perception involves moving from obligations or rules to actual responses and from the particularities of individual experiences to the generalities:

> Perception, we might say, is a process of loving conversation between rules and concrete responses, general conceptions and unique cases, in which the general articulates the particular and is in turn further articulated.

Strategies to promote self-scrutiny or reflection on self

The role of friendship and collegiality have been mentioned in relation to the development of reflection on self or self-scrutiny. Reflective diaries or journals are also becoming a helpful educational strategy in professional education (Banks, 2003). We do not know how Joe and Samina interacted with their colleagues and whether they gained or shared perspectives on their own or others' practice but there seemed to be the potential to do this. This would, of course, have to be managed sensitively. Engaging in self-scrutiny and inviting feedback from friends and colleagues may, on occasion, also require courage and resilience.

Strategies to promote reflection in and on practice

Socratic dialogue (Philippart, 2003) and frameworks for reflection (for example, Boud and Walker, 1998) are helpful in promoting reflection in professional education and practice. The evaluation of reflection is challenging for the ethics educator. Coming to a reasoned conclusion as a result of a process of argument can be demonstrated verbally in student debates and in one-to-one discussions with students. Written accounts may also be assessed. Drawing conclusions about how students reflect in and on practice and on themselves is, however, more difficult. Emphasising to students the inevitability of fallibility and vulnerability of professionals and patients and the importance of honesty seems important.

Strategies to facilitate ethical decision-making

Although they may be criticised as artificial and contrived, some ethical 'decision-making' models or approaches to analysing ethical dilemmas can be useful. They are no substitute for the development of the professional wisdom that comes from experience and from practising the virtues. However, they can help develop skills in the identification of relevant features of a situation, in thinking systemically about values relevant to practice and of potential resources for solutions. One example of a decision-making framework is Goovaerts' (2003) 'staged plan' method, which entails asking a series of questions as follows:

Stage 1: What are the facts?
Stage 2: Whose interests are at stake?
Stage 3: What is the dilemma about?
Stage 4: What are the alternatives?
Stage 5: What is the conclusion?
Stage 6: How to carry out the decision?
Stage 7: Evaluation and reflection.

Professionals and students may find such frameworks helpful in deliberating about practice situations and in helping make decisions (for other examples, see Johnstone, 2004, pp. 108–110; McAuliffe and Chenowith, 2008; David Seedhouse's Values Exchange website, www.values-exchange.com/)

Concluding comments

Professional wisdom involves professionals responding to the nuances and complexity of professional practice, engaging with technical rational and professional artistry views of practice and tolerating the uncertainty and ambiguity of the 'swampy lowland' of everyday professional practice. Professional wisdom comprises perceptual, reflective and decision-making capabilities. It involves professionals seeing the salient features of practice situations, reflecting on self and on the situation, exercising technical and humane judgement and making and acting on decisions.

Professional wisdom is a very necessary virtue guiding and governing the other virtues and encompassing the perceptual and deliberative capabilities that enable professionals to be ethical in practice. Comte-Sponville (2002, p. 31) says that without practical wisdom 'the other virtues are merely good intentions that pave the way to hell'. By association, professional wisdom is the virtue that keeps the virtues on the ethical rails, the development of which enables professionals to aspire to flourishing and to be for the good.

Chapter 5

Care

Introduction

This chapter is concerned with care as a moral quality or virtue. It is a particularly challenging quality to cover, as the term 'care' has many additional meanings (see Brykczyńska, 1997; Morse *et al.*, 1991 for a discussion of concepts of care). For example, we use the terms 'health care' and 'social care' to refer to institutional structures and systems that provide services to look after people's health and social needs and to the practices of the professionals who work in these systems. 'Care' can also be conceptualised as a relationship or an emotion. This means that when practitioners and academics discuss 'care', they may not always be talking about the same concept. Even if we are clear that the focus here is care as a virtue (that is, being a caring kind of person), the connotations associated with the different meanings of care are a background presence and inevitably influence our thinking. The term 'care', like 'community', generally has a positive evaluative meaning associated with warmth, sensitivity and personal engagement. As a practice, it is often associated with women and as a relationship care has been developed as the basis of both feminine and feminist approaches to ethical theory.

After presenting and discussing three vignettes from health and social care settings, this chapter will explore the nature of care, building on the elements of the relationship of care identified by care ethicists and applying this to care as a virtue.

Vignettes

The vignettes that follow depict aspects of professional caring from three different perspectives: a professional social worker (in the role of caregiver); a man who is in hospital (in the role of recipient of care); and a student nurse (in the role of observer and learner). The first vignette is based on an interview with a professional social worker. In the extracts given here, she talks about her orientation to the service users she works with and the importance of thinking about how it feels to be on the receiving end of social work. The second vignette is drawn from research by Morrison (1997) based on interviews with 10 hospital patients asked to talk about their experiences of 'being cared for'. The vignette presented here is based on abstracting some of the information about one of the patients, Tim, from Morrison's overall account. The third vignette is taken from the Royal College of Nursing's (1992) publication based on members' accounts of what they thought was worthwhile about nursing practice. This particular account was given by a nurse, relating to a situation when she was a student being taught how to undertake an uncomfortable procedure with a very sick woman. The student describes the actions and conversation of the woman and the qualified nurse performing the procedure.

1) 'Seeing the client's point of view': comments from Nicola, a hospice social worker

Nicola is a social worker with experience of working in a hospice. She gave a long interview, speaking in great depth about her work. One of the themes that came up frequently was the importance of not being judgemental about people's lifestyles and of trying to see situations from other people's points of view. She commented that she was very keen to take social work students for periods of fieldwork practice:

> The reason that we take a lot of students is to help them to see the other point of view [...] To help them as prospective social workers to see the client's point of view, to see that, to think how it feels to be at the end of social work intervention, to be at the receiving end of it, to be at the receiving end of, in the hospice, medical intervention, to be at the receiving end of [social work].

She then gave an example of what she meant:

> As I said to the Macmillan nurse [specialist nurse for cancer care based at the hospice] one day as she and I were walking up a man's path, I said: 'That man's looking through his window and he must think: "My life has come to this, here I am and there's a social worker and a nurse coming up my path"'. You can't get much worse than that in life really because what it says, it says something about that man's life. It says on every level he's having to resort to this support and it's a long way from a man who once thought he was independent, a person who was in control of his own life. One of them says: 'You're dying' and the other one says 'You're not coping socially'. And you know, if you look at it in terms of how he felt about that, that must have been such a deeply depressing thing for him to see coming up his path, this bevy of people who were saying 'You need lots of help here on every level'; and for somebody who's not used to that, extraordinarily undermining. And I have to know that my presence is not always welcomed. I may think that I'm supporting people but what they see when a social worker turns up is something quite different [they think]: 'I've failed'.
> (Source: interview)

2) Tim's experience in hospital

Tim is a 48-year-old man who had been a patient in a ward of a large teaching hospital for several weeks. When he was in hospital he discovered he had lung cancer and had spent a period of time feeling very anxious about his condition and prognosis. He had been transferred to another hospital for a series of diagnostic investigations, which were long and drawn out and experienced by Tim as very traumatic. His condition was complicated by high blood pressure, which had necessitated his move to the other hospital for specialist care. He reported having a very positive experience when he returned to the ward in the original hospital – the nurses were genuinely glad to see him return:

> When they seen me come back here last week, young Jane got hold of me as if she hadn't seen me for donkey's years, as if I was a long lost brother or something. They made me feel like somebody.

Tim was described by the researcher as 'an extremely nervous patient'. The nurses' ability to calm Tim when he was a very anxious patient, without resorting to the use of tranquillisers, was important. Tim himself commented that there was no 'front' to the nurses' attitude, and that they always displayed a concern 'for his well-being' and it was a genuine concern.
(Source: Adapted from Morrison, 1997, pp. 107, 108, 110, 116, 119)

3) A student nurse's observation

I was being taught by the enrolled nurse how to pass a nasogastric tube[1] on a patient. The lady we were working on was quite poorly. She had lung cancer and had had fluid drained from her pleural cavity twice that week [...] The enrolled nurse explained to her exactly what we were going to do and how much better she would feel. He was quite clear about how unpleasant the tube could be when it was going over the back of her throat. He then explained it again to me and she watched like a hawk, holding the tube he had given her in her hand. After all the preparation, he proceeded to put the tube up to her nose, and lifted her two hands and wrapped them round his. 'At any time when you want you can stop this,' he said. So she did, three seconds later. The second time, he was just as patient. Eventually, with tears pouring down her face, she pushed at his hand to 'help' the tube going right down her throat. After she was all tidied up and settled, and some of the bile had been drained off, we all held hands for a second, and he made her laugh by inviting her to help with the intubation of any other patient who might need it.
(Source: Royal College of Nursing, 1992, quoted in Davies,1998, p. 127)

Reflections

The first vignette differs from the others in that it does not just give an account of a particular situation or event where a moral quality (in this case, caring) was exhibited. Nicola, the social worker, first

---

[1] A tube inserted through the nose to drain the stomach.

expresses a view about what makes a good social worker – being non-judgemental and seeing situations from the point of view of others. She obviously thinks this is important as she expresses a keenness to develop this capacity in students. The particular situation she then describes is not her actual face-to-face meeting with the man she is going to visit, but rather what she is thinking and saying to her colleague prior to the meeting. Her thoughts focus on what she imagines the man might be thinking and feeling as he watches a nurse and a social worker walking up his path.

Nicola has not met the man – her only connection with him is the face looking through the window. She is not paying attention to his viewpoint or needs in particular (she does not know these yet), but she is indicating that already she is in an empathic frame of mind, she is using her *moral imagination* – she is open and ready to meet this man and to listen and respond to him. She is aware of the potential impact of the presence of herself and the nurse on the man. We have included this example specifically because it is not based on an account of an activity, but more an *initial orientation*, a preparation for a first encounter. Nicola is giving an account of herself as a certain kind of person – arguably a professional who cares about the people she works with. She is preparing herself to act as a caring person in the meeting with the man.

The second vignette is from the perspective of someone 'on the receiving end' (of nursing care). A man in hospital, Tim, gives an account of how the nurses welcomed him on his return to the ward. He talks about their emotional response to him, rather than the administration of medicines or the ministering to his bodily needs. His description of the young nurse, Jane, getting hold of him 'as if I was a long lost brother' suggests a physical embrace and a personalised response. His comment: 'They made me feel like somebody' indicates that he felt they genuinely cared about him. This might be contrasted with being treated like nobody (ignored) or anybody (given a standard treatment, rather than singled out as a special person). Tim's account focuses on the *emotional* aspect of the caring relationship he has with the nurses. In this case, unlike the first one, a *relationship* has developed between the nurses and Tim, which means they not only know him (including how to calm him) but also seem to regard him with affection. Tim's use of the analogy of himself as Jane's 'long lost brother' draws attention to the nature of the caring being offered by the nurses as similar in quality to that of a family.

The final account is given by a third party who has been observing an experienced nurse. This time a medical procedure is being carried out and the focus of the description is very much on the *activity* that takes place. The description does not include the thoughts and feelings of the person giving the account (as in Tim's story), nor does the student impute any thoughts or feelings to other participants (as Nicola does in the first vignette). What is given is a description of an activity that involves the nurse communicating with the woman (explaining the procedure); giving her a means to have some control over what he is doing (by stopping his hands); inserting a tube; allowing her to stop the procedure and waiting patiently; successfully inserting the tube and draining the bile; holding hands; and making the woman laugh. Apart from describing the nurse as 'patient', the student does not use any other emotional or evaluative terms in her description of what the nurse did. Yet what he did was clearly much more than simply inserting a tube and draining bile and the descriptions the student gives highlight what the student thought was significant in the way the nurse performed the task. He initiated a relationship with the woman that was caring and empowering. By placing her hands over his, he not only gave her the power to stop his actions directly (rather than indirectly by making a noise), but he also put her in physical contact with him. This import of this gesture was reinforced by all three participants holding hands afterwards, signifying, perhaps, a recognition that they had been jointly involved in a difficult exercise.

The way this account of a nursing procedure performed with care is written is also of interest. The student was an observer, but an engaged observer. The student was there to learn. The close description given by the student of the key features of the activity focuses on what the experienced nurse did to develop a relationship with the woman. The student was metaphorically 'walking alongside' both parties and could probably be described as 'emotionally engaged' (the handholding at the end suggests this). She was being attentive, sensitive and perceptive – picking up on the ethically significant aspects of the activity.

Care as a virtue and care as a relation

The vignettes discussed above were chosen as examples of the kinds of attitudes, approaches and actions we might expect of professional practitioners we would describe as exhibiting the moral quality of 'caring'. Care is not one of the traditional virtues identified by

Aristotle or Aquinas, but it has resonances with Hume's concept of sympathy (Hume, 1739/1960) and has been identified as an important moral virtue by several recent theorists (Gastmans, 2006; Slote, 2001; Van Hooft, 2006b). For some care is the cardinal or basic virtue from which all others follow (Slote, 2001), for others it is one virtue amongst many (Timmons, 2002).

Discussion of care as a virtue is complicated by the fact that in recent years a specific ethical theory or approach to ethics known as the ethic(s) of care has been developed that focuses on the primacy of caring. This approach has some commonalities with virtue ethics, including a rejection of the principle- and rationality-based approaches to ethics of deontology and consequentialism. Yet while some theorists see care ethics as a version of virtue ethics (Boss, 1998, pp. 398–406; McLaren, 2001; Timmons, 2002, pp. 224–232), others explicitly do not (Held, 2006, pp. 19–20; Noddings, 2002, pp. 19–21). According to Noddings, one of the leading exponents of the ethics of care, care ethics has a special focus on the recipient of care, and the relationship between the carer and person being cared for. In virtue ethics, the focus of attention is on the person caring. So for care ethicists who see care primarily in terms of a relationship, to regard care as a virtue of the person who cares is only a partial picture. Let us now examine what might be the components of care, to enable us to assess which aspects might be construed as comprising the virtue of care.

Elements of care

Exponents of the ethics of care have been concerned to develop a rich and nuanced picture of the nature of caring. The literature in this field has burgeoned in recent decades, following the early seminal work of moral psychologist Gilligan (1982) and philosopher of education Noddings (1984), who were concerned to show that there were alternative moral voices or approaches to ethics than those that prioritised principles and rational argument. Not surprisingly, the care approach has become increasingly popular in the ethics literature of the 'caring professions', particularly in nursing (Bowden, 1997, pp. 101–140; Bradshaw, 1996; Fry, 1989; Hanford, 1994; Tschudin, 2003), and more recently in social work (Banks, 2004, pp. 89–92; Clifford, 2002; Hugman, 2005, pp. 67–85; Parton, 2003). There are many and varied accounts of the nature of caring. One of the most influential is the analysis of the elements of care offered by Tronto (1993), which has been used by moral philosophers, social policy theorists and those interested in professional ethics in nursing and social work, including theorists who have developed an account of care as a virtue (for example, Gastmans, 2006, pp. 136–137). Tronto identifies four elements of care, along with 'integrity', which she argues holds all the elements together (1993, pp. 127–136). We will summarise these, illustrating with reference to the three vignettes.

Attentiveness

This feature of care is often termed *caring about*, that is, noticing the need for care in the first place; actively seeking awareness of others and their needs and points of view. This can be personal or impersonal, depending on whether we are paying attention to a particular individual person known to us, particular people unknown to us, hypothetical people or human- or animal-kind in general. Nicola, the social worker in the first vignette, could be said to display an impersonal attentiveness to the needs of social work service users in general, and a semi-personal attentiveness to the potential needs of a man she had seen but not met. The way the experienced nurse in the third vignette treated the woman while he was inserting the tube (his patience, the touching of hands) suggests that he was very attentive to her personal needs and feelings. This dimension of care includes people's motives (the desire to meet people's needs), and what has been called moral sensitivity – awareness of how our actions affect others (Rest, 1994, p. 22). This is very similar to what Vetlesen (1994, p. 6) calls *moral perception* (see also Blum, 1994), which involves the use of the faculty of *empathy* (a disposition to develop concern for others) to see the morally relevant features of a situation ('the features that carry importance for the weal and woe of human beings involved').

Responsibility

This element of care has sometimes been designated as *taking care of*, that is, assuming responsibility for care – with responsibility being embedded in a set of implicit cultural practices (rather than a set of formal rules or series of promises). The assumption of responsibility may be based on a number of factors (we may have contributed to the need for care, we may have a special relationship that entails a caring responsibility or we may simply recognise a need for caring). This responsibility may or may not involve actually carrying out any of the tasks of caring. For example, Nicola, the social worker, clearly presents herself as taking responsibility for improving the condition of the people she works with. This responsibility is part of her professional role. Before she even meets the man and does any of the actual work of care, she is taking responsibility for meeting his needs and anticipating her contribution to causing him concern or unease.

Competence

This is about *care-giving*, the actual work of care that needs to be done – one's ability to do something about another's needs. The term 'competence' is being used here in an holistic sense relating to professionals' abilities and capacities, rather than a set of discrete technical skills (competencies). Tronto (1993, p. 133) says she includes competence as a moral dimension of care to avoid the bad faith of people who will 'take care of' a problem without being willing to engage in care-giving. She comments that is it especially important that competence is regarded as being part of professional ethics, so that 'we would not permit individuals to escape from responsibility for their incompetence by claiming to adhere to a code of professional ethics' (p. 134). The description of the way the experienced nurse in the third vignette carried out the tube insertion is a good example of the integration of ethical treatment and practical competence, involving gaining informed consent, promoting patient choice and dignity and accomplishing a technical procedure (inserting a tube and draining bile). It might be said that, as discussed in Chapter 4, the nurse was combining technical rational competence with professional artistry. The nurses looking after Tim in the second vignette are described as being able to calm him without resorting to tranquillisers. That suggests a degree of competence, with their actions stemming from their sense of responsibility to meet his needs in the best possible way and their attentiveness (noticing, listening, empathic concern) to his anxieties and behaviour.

Responsiveness

The focus here is on *care-receiving*, the response of that which is cared for to the care. Tronto (1993, p. 135) regards this feature of care as vitally important, as it is a reminder of the inequalities that exist in society and the dangers faced by people who are vulnerable at the hands of their care-givers. This suggests the need to keep a balance between the needs of givers and receivers of care. Tronto argues that this is not the same as reciprocity. Responsiveness suggests we consider the position of others as they express it. Again the experienced nurse inserting the tube displayed this feature, particularly exemplified in his willingness to go at the pace determined by the woman. Tim's comments about the nurses' treatment of him during his hospital stay suggested he responded positively to their attitudes and actions, especially appreciating being treated personally, as someone special. Those receiving care may not always respond, but it is important to regard them as potentially responsive.

The integrity of care

According to Tronto (1993, pp. 136–137), good care requires that the four elements or phases fit together as a whole, which involves knowledge of the context of the care process and making judgements about conflicting needs and strategies. These judgements include assessment of needs in a social and political as well as personal context. For Tronto, this last point is very important, as she wants to develop care as a political ideal, based on the notion that all humans need care – challenging the separation of private and public life. The dimensions of care outlined above should not, she claims, be restricted to the immediate objects of our care, but can also inform our practices as citizens (p. 168). This fifth element of care suggests to us the need for professional wisdom in making judgements and assessments carefully, sensitively and in the light of the relevant social and political context.

As Gastmans (2006, p. 137) points out, these dimensions of care indicate that 'good care demands more than just good intention; good care should be understood as the practice of combining activities, attitudes and knowledge of the situation'. Assuming we work with Tronto's account of care as a relationship, we will now consider which of these dimensions of care are present in care as a virtue. Noddings and Held, in their critiques of care as a virtue, appear to regard virtue ethics as focusing largely on Tronto's first dimension, attentiveness or 'caring about'. Noddings (2002, p. 21) claims, 'It is entirely possible for an individual, exercising a host of recognised virtues, to care sincerely (in the virtue sense) and yet not connect with the recipient of care'. Held (2006, p. 20) offers a similar critique, suggesting that caring as a virtue may neglect the labour involved and objective results of caring (that is, what Tronto identifies as competence and responsiveness). Held argues that caring is 'not only a question of motive or attitude or virtue' (what Tronto calls attentiveness). These critiques of care as a virtue are based on a rather limited view of the nature of a virtue as primarily to do with motives and attitudes (attentiveness).

The professional virtue of caring

If we regard virtue as more than simply an 'inner state' or motive, then we may be able to offer an account of care as a virtue, that is, 'being caring', that covers all Tronto's dimensions. We have already suggested in Chapter 3 that many virtues could be described as 'relational virtues' or 'other-regarding'. That is, they are defined (or are frequently defined) in relation to other people: for example, care, trustworthiness, justice and respectfulness (when applied to people). Others, like courage, integrity or the Aristotelian virtue of temperance, have less of a relational quality.

Van Hooft (2006a; 2006b), developing the analysis of Audi (1997), outlines eight features of virtuous action, which include not only the agent's motivation, but the agent's knowledge and understanding of the field of the virtue and consideration of the beneficiaries of the virtue. Van Hooft (2006b, p. 59) argues that the virtue of caring 'embraces all aspects of action, including the emotions, motivations, knowledge and ethical thinking that enter into it'. Van Hooft (2006b, p. 60) discusses caring as a core virtue in nursing in some depth and offers a definition of the virtue of caring as:

> The comportment of self towards others which has the inherent goal of enhancing the existence of those others – whether they are others in intimate relation to me, others for whom I have professional responsibility, or others with whom I identify simply because they are compatriots, co-religionists or fellow members of the human race.

In the context of nursing the inherent goal (what we called the core purpose or 'service ideal' in our discussion in Chapter 2) is enhancing the health-related existence of those others for whom the nurse has professional responsibility. If we were to apply this to social work, then the goal would be the enhancement of social welfare.

Let us explore Noddings' suggestion that a person may care sincerely in the virtue sense, yet not connect with the recipient of care. By 'connect' we include use of moral imagination or empathy to relate to people who are far away and whom we may never meet. What would we say about someone we might describe as a 'caring' and morally admirable person, who did not connect with the people she cared about? If part of what being caring comprises is the ability to connect, then in this instance we might say that what was happening was not caring (in that sense). If we take the example of Nicola, featured in the first vignette, based on the information given in the vignette, we might say, 'Nicola is a very caring person', meaning she is generally empathic, competent and responsible. Yet let us assume that she went into the man's house, met him and was unable to connect with him. Let us say he found her too intense, overly concerned and patronising. If Nicola is as sensitive and skilled as she claims, she may pull back in response to the man's initial reaction and change her approach. But she may still fail to connect, assuming that by connecting we mean reaching the man in a positive way. If Nicola did all we would expect a caring person to do in these circumstances and the man still failed to respond, we might not blame Nicola, who after all is a caring person (both in terms of her attitude and competence in care-giving). Rather we might regard the man as resistant, depressed, awkward or simply unresponsive in some way. On the other hand, if Nicola repeatedly fails to connect with the people she visits, then we might review our description of her as 'caring'. If caring is about connecting, then someone who repeatedly fails to connect would not be regarded as caring. This requires us to describe the virtue of care as more than just 'caring about'. We may or may not regard this as acceptable, depending on how we see a virtue. If a virtue is a motive or emotion, and is agent-based as Slote argues, then care as a virtue would simply comprise 'caring about' and the criticisms made by Noddings and Held would seem to be legitimate. However, if we adopt a more expansive account of the nature of the virtues as presented in Chapters 2 and 3, this gives a place to the labour involved in exhibiting a virtue and the experiences of the people on the receiving end (if the virtue is a relational virtue).

Understanding the virtue of care as involving creative struggle to maintain a balance (Aristotle's concept of a 'mean') between smothering/excessive concern and indifference may be helpful here. The person with a caring motive and failing to connect may be overwhelming, or smothering. The person without a caring motive, but who is competent at performing basic 'caring' roles may veer more towards indifference. Care as a professional virtue, we would argue, comprises a motive of attentiveness towards particular others for whom the professional takes responsibility, and competence in care-giving, tailored to the responses of the person cared for. This might be regarded as the full account of caring. If we consider virtues as modular in the way described in Chapter 3, then it might be plausible to regard Tronto's elements of care as modules – some of which can exist independently of the whole package ('full' or 'composite' caring).

Strategies for practice and professional education

Assuming caring to entail the elements of attentiveness, responsibility, competence, responsiveness of the cared for and a kind of integrity in bringing all this together, we will now consider how this moral quality (or these modules) can be developed in health and social care practitioners.

Developing moral perception and sensitivity through observations

Tronto's first element of care, attentiveness, is about focusing on the other person – listening, looking, 'feeling with' and 'connecting with' the other. Noddings (1984, p. 30) explicitly distinguishes 'feeling with' from empathy (putting oneself in the other's shoes). She describes caring as 'receiving the other into myself' or what she calls 'engrossment' (p. 33). This requires developing skills in observing, listening, focusing and attending – as clearly exemplified in the third vignette about the nurse inserting a naso-gastric tube while the student was an engaged observer. Carefully observing a patient or service user whilst another practitioner works with them is a good way of developing these skills. The next stage for the student nurse will be to insert a tube herself. And whilst she will certainly focus on ensuring that the tube is inserted correctly, this student nurse will probably also attempt to connect with her patient in the same way she observed in the experienced nurse. Watching video material and discussing in class the dynamics of the interactions between service users and practitioners is also a useful strategy.

Role playing, discussing scenarios and real-life rehearsal

The opportunity to act out the role of the person on the receiving end of care in a scenario is also a good way of feeling what it might be like to be in this position. Various scenarios could be used involving the carer being over-concerned, barely competent, highly competent but disengaged and attempting to be the 'ideal carer'. On completing the scenarios, mutual feedback can be given by each participant to the other, which helps with learning – as well as engaging the audience, if a group of people have been watching. For developing competence in various caring practices that require technical skills as well as a particular attitude or orientation, then the opportunity actually to practise doing these tasks whilst being observed and supervised by an experienced practitioner is invaluable, as is the opportunity to reflect afterwards on what went well, badly and what improvements could be made next time. Sometimes it is possible, with the permission of all parties involved, to video-record a trainee practitioner undertaking a procedure or an interview. This gives very valuable material for learning in class, supervision or team meetings.

Role modelling

As shown in the vignette featuring the student nurse, the experienced nurse was not just giving a technical demonstration but was also serving as a role model for excellent practice. The fact that this scene was remembered suggests how significant it was at the time, and probably has been in the development of that former student nurse as a caring and competent practitioner. Having available role models for good service user/patient care is vitally important, as is the modelling of caring behaviour of senior practitioners towards trainees or less experienced practitioners.

Developing a caring organisational ethos

Whilst not wanting to 'over protect' staff or patients/service users, or to create an overly 'friendly' or informal atmosphere, clearly it is important for an organisation, team or unit to develop and maintain an ethos where attentiveness, responsiveness and highly competent care-giving are the norm. This will be mutually reinforcing if staff care for and about each other as well as patients/service users, if they prioritise care-giving above other demands (such as quick turnover or resource-saving measures) and the relevant targets, paperwork and rewards reflect this too. Tim's account of his experience of being in a hospital ward in the second vignette seems to capture a warm and caring ethos in the ward.

Concluding comments

We have followed Tronto's analysis of care as entailing attentiveness, responsibility, competence, responsiveness of the person cared-for and a certain kind of integrity in bringing these elements together with an awareness of the relevant social and political context. While Tronto and care ethicists see care as a relation, we have argued that care can also be seen as a virtue (being caring), and as such is a relational virtue, as it requires a degree of engagement between the carer and the person/people being cared for. We would hesitate to call a practitioner 'caring' if they were well motivated to give good quality care to an individual or set of people, yet were not competent either technically or in terms of their communication skills to do so. However, as with the other virtues, care can be regarded as modular, with some practitioners having a disposition to be caring in some situations and not others. Practitioners may also be regarded as 'good enough' at caring or relatively caring, whilst the virtue of 'full caring' remains an ideal to be aspired towards.

Chapter 6

Respectfulness

Introduction[1]

The term 'respect' is much referred to in everyday conversation. People talk of earning and showing respect and also, in language of the street, of 'dissing' (meaning showing disrespect). Respect appears in professional codes as 'respect for' a range of value objects, for example, respect for persons, privacy, dignity, autonomy and confidentiality. In moral philosophy, 'respect for persons' is expressed as a fundamental principle with the potential to include or exclude individuals from ethical consideration. Lack of respect also makes headlines in health and social care services when people's dignity, privacy and autonomy are violated. What respectfulness requires of professionals in their everyday practice is generally not made explicit. In this chapter we move beyond rhetorical references to respect and reclaim respectfulness as a meaningful professional virtue, focusing on its positive attributes and implications.

We consider examples of respect from health and social care and distinguish amongst different types of respect, most significantly between recognition respect and appraisal respect, as outlined by Darwell, and between respect for others and self-respect. Building on the work of Joseph Raz, we suggest a continuum or four-stage process of respect that may be demonstrated by the respectful practitioner. This comprises acknowledgement,

---

[1] Some of the material in this chapter draws on an unpublished PhD thesis (Gallagher 2003).

preservation, non-destruction and engagement. We discuss the nature of respectfulness as a virtue, which, in an Aristotelian sense, would lie between the extremes of servility or sycophancy and disrespect.

Vignettes

There are many possible examples of respect and disrespect within health and social care practice and here we have selected two. The first is from an interview with Debbie, a social worker, who works with vulnerable families. The second is from an interview with Ming-Li, a nurse researcher who has conducted research with older people from the Chinese community in Britain. The examples are quite different, suggesting the complexity and ambiguity of everyday professional practice, the relationship between respect and culture and also the significance of respectful relationships not just between service users, their families and professionals but also between professionals.

1) 'That basic respect': A social worker's perspective

Debbie is a social worker, based in a Children's Centre offering support to vulnerable children and families. She gave an account of her work with a particular family in the course of an interview. She describes the family as 'chaotic'. The mother, Lorraine, struggles with her drug addiction and her five-year-old son, Jimmy, is often late for school. Debbie has been working with Lorraine encouraging her to build constructive relationships with school staff. In response to this she tells Debbie that she feels unable to do this.

> [Lorraine said] 'Every time I walk into that school they look at me like I'm a drug user.' And so I tried to help her unpick things. I [Debbie] said: 'How do you mean? Is it just that you're very aware that you are?' And I really tried and I felt awful afterwards because I worked very hard with her to try and get her to think that all they were worried about was Jimmy getting to school on time; and how important his education is; and that it is his right, and that it is Lorraine's legal responsibility, to get him there. I said: 'Maybe they're not looking at you as a drug user'. And she said: 'You wouldn't understand anything about it'.

Debbie explained how she attended a meeting at the school to discuss children of concern. She noticed that Jimmy was not on the list.

So they [the teachers] said: 'Any other business?' And I said: 'I just wondered how Jimmy was getting on?' And the teacher and the learning mentor worker said: 'Oh, that woman!' And I thought: 'I asked about a child called Jimmy here'. And the teacher said: 'She's such a waster, she's just a complete drug addict', and almost spat. I mean her body language was just disgusting. And I said: 'And how's Jimmy?' But she couldn't [respond]. And I said: 'I really have to challenge you on what you've just done'. And I said: 'I've been working very hard with mum who said she felt judged every time she came in the school. And I was trying to say: "No, no, no, Lorraine, you aren't, you aren't, you aren't"'. And I said: 'Now I know that I owe her an apology, because I've just seen what she feels every time she comes in here'. The teacher got very defensive and I said: 'We need to change the way we think about people'. And I explained what that start point was, because I said: 'You still haven't said how Jimmy is, that was my question. I know how mum is because I work closely with her'. So the whole meeting then became about that and about how such judgements impact on the way you see people, because you're seeing Jimmy as the child of a drug addict, not Jimmy the five-year-old who has a right to an education and who's battling with chaotic parents, etcetera, etcetera.

Debbie said that she had not wanted her intervention to be a 'personal attack' against the teacher but felt strongly that she needed to 'make the point'. After the meeting the teacher followed her out of the school to apologise and thank her. Debbie reported that she said to the teacher:

'Well I would be happy to have more conversations on that level'. And so for a while we kind of introduced the topic of values into the school meetings, just for a while. Obviously I didn't tell Lorraine about that conversation and then I asked her a week or so later: 'How are you getting on with school?' She said: 'God, it's so different, you know I've been invited in at the end of school now, each day now I go in and just have five minutes feedback with the teacher'. And I said: 'How does that feel?' She said: 'It's great, and so now I know what he's doing in school and we do it together and if I've got a worry about his behaviour at home

I speak to the teacher'. Lorraine never knew what the catalyst, the change had been, and I don't suppose for one minute, because not all the teachers are there at the meeting obviously, it's just a choice few teachers. But that to me spoke a lot. And, you know, I could give other, similar examples of that basic respect, which underpins everything we do in social work.

(Source: interview)

2) Respect and culture: the view of a nurse researcher

The second example comes from an interview with Ming-Li, a nurse researcher, who was born in China and then moved to Hong Kong before coming to Britain to become a nurse. The interview focused on the relationship between respect and culture in relation to Ming-Li's work as a nurse and as a researcher. She described her own culture as 'traditionally Chinese' and herself as 'a modern, educated woman'. Ming-Li talked of respect as the 'mainstay in our lives' with origins in the philosophy of Confucius. She defined respect as follows:

It's to treat the person as a person in their own right, you know, equality. I'm equal to you and you're equal to me and you don't tell me what to do, I make my own decisions. I'm able to make my own decisions and you ought to respect my decisions whether it's bad or good. I mean you can give opinions but whether I accept it or not that should be respected and to me it has something to do with age as well. I've learnt to or I wanted to respect people who are older, like my parents, my grandparents. So that's familial and also those people who are senior to me because in Hong Kong culture we were taught at school that we had to respect our teachers, your headmasters and you do not ask questions or challenge your teachers. So that seniority was what we were told to respect. I think basically it's underpinned by humanity.

In her early practice, Ming-Li worked as a nurse working with people with learning disabilities. She shared her experience of working in institutionalised cultures in Britain in the 1960s that she considered disrespectful and dehumanising. She described the approach as 'just routine and the residents, called patients then, with learning disabilities were just treated like, to me, it felt like treating them like a flock of birds, of animals, chickens, you know, in and out. It was matter of fact, there was no human touch'. She gave the following example:

Everybody had the same tea, everyone had sugar in the tea. It didn't occur to us that we had to ask: 'What would you like?' We just took it for granted that they didn't understand us.

In relation to her current practice as a nurse researcher, Ming-Li emphasised the relationship between respect, biography and culture. She talked about how she demonstrates respect in her research practice as she interviews older Chinese people:

The residents speak different Chinese languages. Because of my upbringing I was told that, you know, you please people and respect people by trying to speak in their own language so I did try [...] I do not take it for granted that I'm a researcher and therefore I'm very powerful. I didn't go in with that view. I treated them as my grandmothers, my mother, you know that seniority of respect [...] If they tell me to sit in that corner, I do and also ask for permission if I could ask questions around that area each time. Although they have given me permission, on paper, they signed it but I find that as a researcher consent is not a fixed category, you have to negotiate every minute during your interview especially when you are asking touchy questions in relation to the relationship with the family [...] When they volunteer questions like that I had to be very careful [regarding] what I would like to ask as the next question. I had to ask: 'Is this alright?' I also realised that because the interview time was around lunch-time, I would say: 'Oh, I'm so sorry would you like me to leave you to have your dinner?' They would say: 'No, no that's alright.' They wanted to talk because they had nobody to talk to as long as I have done with them. So, yes, I was very aware of respecting that person, that elderly person, that could have been my grandmother, my mother, my parents. So with that view, that's the kind of respect underpinned by seniority, my culture, my upbringing, you know.
(Source: interview)

Reflections

In the first example the social worker, Debbie, begins by referring to this 'chaotic family' with whom she is working. She had been working particularly hard with the mother, Lorraine, encouraging her to build positive relationships with the school staff. Debbie was, it seems, trying to get Lorraine to accept that the concern of school staff was about Jimmy getting to school on time and his right to an education. She did not appear to believe that the teachers might be prejudiced against Lorraine nor that they might exclude her. It was only when Debbie asked about Jimmy at the school meeting that she came to realise that at least one teacher had extremely negative and strong views. Both the teacher's response ('almost spat') and Debbie's analysis ('just disgusting') appear visceral and emotional. Emotions are often not made explicit in discussions of professional ethics. It seems possible that whereas the teacher's response may reflect prejudice and perhaps ignorance, Debbie gives an account of her response as based on her sense of 'that basic respect that underpins everything that we do in social work'. Debbie also represents herself as being respectful towards the teacher ('I didn't want it to be a personal attack'). Although we have used this vignette to explore respectfulness, clearly other virtues also seem relevant to Debbie's account, for example, courage, trustworthiness, integrity and professional wisdom.

In the second example derived from an interview with Ming-Li, a nurse researcher, the relationship between respect and culture is explored. Ming-Li discusses culture in different ways: in relation to her Chinese identity; in relation to institutionalised cultures of care in the 1960s; and in relation to her work as a nurse researcher engaged in research with older people from Chinese communities. Ming-Li emphasises how respect is integral to Chinese culture ('the mainstay') particularly in relation to older people and those in professional roles such as teaching. Ming-Li shares her experience of disrespectful institutional cultures where people with learning disabilities were denied individualised care or the 'human touch' and treated, rather, as 'flocks of birds'.

In her research practice, Ming-Li appears to strike a balance between, at least, two cultures. She describes herself as a Western, educated woman and also as traditionally Chinese. She represents herself as respectful of the culture and seniority of the older Chinese participants using, where possible, their language and sitting where she is advised to sit. She also refers to consent to research participation acknowledging that signing the consent form is just part of the process. She states that this has to be negotiated as the interview progresses. Ming-Li's sensitivity and respectfulness towards the older Chinese participants is likely to have been informed by her cultural awareness and cultural and ethical values.

Respect[2]

Before discussing respectfulness as a virtue, we will spend some time exploring the nature of respect as a concept. The term 'respect' comes from the Latin *respicere* translated as 'to look back' or 'to look again', to 're-spect'. This suggests that respect is an evaluating concept that involves appraising or looking over. To respect something requires some activity and is therefore active rather than passive. Dillon (2005) offers a particularly helpful explanation:

> Respect is, most generally, a relation between a subject and an object, in which the subject responds to the object from a certain perspective in some appropriate way. Respect necessarily has an object: respect is always for, directed toward, paid to, felt about, shown for some object. While a wide variety of things can be appropriate objects of one kind of respect or another, the subject of respect is always a person, that is, a conscious rational being capable of recognizing things, being self-consciously and intentionally responsive to them, and having and expressing values with regard to them.

This account of respect focusing on the relationship between subjects and objects is a helpful lynchpin in our understanding of respect. Health and social care professionals are both subjects and objects of respect. They are self-conscious, rational (for the most part) and are able to recognise and respond to objects of value. From the perspectives of other colleagues and, perhaps, service users and society more generally they may also be objects of respect.

The professional codes of health and social care professionals (for example, General Medical Council, 2006; General Social Care Council, 2004; Nursing & Midwifery Council, 2008) point to a range of objects that professionals should respect, for example, individuality, autonomy, dignity, confidentiality, privacy, rights and the values and responsibilities within the code. The meaning of, distinction between, and means to arbitrate amongst these different objects of respect within codes is not made explicit. If asked, Debbie may have said that she acted in the way she did because she respects the

---

[2] This section is based on material drawn from a previously published article: Gallagher, A. (2007) 'The respectful nurse', *Nursing Ethics*, vol. 14, no. 3, pp. 360–371.

individuality, autonomy or dignity of service users. Perhaps, she is also keen to promote the self-respect of service users. Ming-Li, in her account, emphasises the significance of respect for older people and for those in certain positions.

Types of respect

Respect is both self-regarding (self-respect) and other-regarding (respect for). It relates to the way we think, feel and act towards ourselves and the thoughts, feelings and actions we have in relation to others. Both dimensions are relevant to health and social care. Professionals need to have a sense of self-respect and need to aspire to maintaining and developing this in others. They also need to have some sense of what 'respect for' others means and involves, particularly as there are so many, sometimes competing, objects of respect.

'Recognition respect' and 'appraisal respect' are two types of respect outlined by Darwell (1995). The former allows that something is worthy of respect. It is recognised that this is the kind of thing that is an appropriate object of respect. Humans, it can be argued, are worthy of respect in this sense and this is not a matter of degree. People are to be respected equally in all circumstances. Appraisal respect allows that there are differences in the amount of respect we bestow on objects based on the appraisal of certain qualities. Middleton (2006, p. 63) summarises these types of respect as follows:

> Recognition respect is not concerned with appraising in anything other than a broad sense – is this object the type of object that can be respected? Appraisal respect tells us that the answer to that question is positive and leaves us the possibility of placing the object on some continuum.

Recognition respect and appraisal respect are relevant to the way people see each other. In everyday and professional encounters, the respect-worthiness of others is both recognised and appraised and the responses are tailored appropriately. Whereas recognition respect is not a matter of degree or individual discernment, appraisal respect involves judgement based on some set of criteria. When people behave in ethically exemplary ways, for example, they may be appraised as deserving of a high degree of respect, whereas those who perform minimally may be appraised as deserving of less respect.

Middleton adapts and extends Darwell's typology of respect for others to self-respect, distinguishing between human self-respect, appraisal self-respect and status self-respect. Human self-respect requires recognition of our own sense of worth as humans and is not reliant on the responses of others. Middleton (2006, p. 66) says,

Self-respect is not simply a reflection of the respect we receive from others, although of course that is important. It is also about how we feel about ourselves. It is partly about maintaining a set of standards. These standards allow us to construct ourselves as persons worth respecting.

Appraisal self-respect relates to 'the way we celebrate the person we are. Not to others, but to ourselves.' Such self-respect goes beyond recognising that we are of worth but is also about having pride in achievements. Status self-respect emerges from recognition of our role in society by having a title or position ('Dean', 'President' or 'Chief Executive', for example) or belonging to a group such as a cultural or professional group.

Self-respect is an important contributory factor to human flourishing. Rawls (1971, p. 440) describes an individual's self-respect as 'perhaps the most important primary good' and as having two aspects:

It includes a sense of his [sic] own value, his secure conviction that his conception of the good, his plan of life, is worth carrying out. And secondly, self-respect implies a confidence in one's ability, so far as it is within one's power, to fulfil one's intentions [...] . Without it nothing may seem worth doing, or if some things have value for us, we lack the will to strive for them. All desire and activity becomes empty and vain and we sink into apathy and cynicism.

For professionals, self-respect relates very much to their sense of the value of their practice and to a sense that what they are doing is worthwhile. Aspiring to a set of professional values and a regulatory service ideal will be part of that. For service users, self-respect is important in their having a sense of a worthwhile life. A lack of self-respect, for professionals and service users, has the potential to thwart their sense of purpose and motivation. The respect shown to or withheld from us by others has the potential to enhance or diminish our self-respect and it seems plausible that our ability to demonstrate respect for others is influenced by our sense of self-respect.

Consideration of the implications of self-respect, therefore, highlights some of the features of human vulnerability and dependency discussed in Chapter 1. As Middleton (2006, p.65) says,

> The way others treat us can clearly affect our self-respect. But, if others' treatment constituted our self-respect we would become dependent upon others' actions toward us. But the construction of self-respect is not simply a reflection of others' respect for us.

It is interesting to note, therefore, that many of the things that contribute to our self-respect may remain hidden to others, privileged to us. Others cannot always know our intentions, motivations, inner struggles or sacrifices and part of self-respect may be about precisely that – keeping to ourselves the thoughts and feelings that support self-respect.

Respect and self-respect apply to professionals and service users alike and they are thus important for ethical professional practice. This involves respecting dignity and autonomy and also supporting and developing self-respect. Professionals require self-respect and must also demonstrate respect for others of the three types outlined above: by recognising the respect-worthiness of everyone as humans; by valuing achievements and capabilities; and by recognising status and valuing the groups to which people belong.

Returning to the examples of Debbie and Ming-Li, it seems possible to apply Middleton's types of respect. Both appear to recognise the humanity of other people. Debbie acknowledges the achievements of those who use services even if their lives are 'chaotic' and they are initially lacking in motivation to change. She also recognises the status of those she works with, for example other professionals, but she is not unduly deferential. Debbie challenges the negative and disrespectful attitude of a teacher colleague. Ming-Li points to disrespectful care of people with learning disabilities in the 1960s when, it appears, they were excluded from moral consideration, being neither recognised nor appraised as worthy of respect. Their care lacked humanity or the 'human touch' and they were, according to Ming-Li, treated as less than human and more like birds or animals. Since this time there has been a radical shift in the philosophy of care in relation to people with learning disabilities. There is now a focus on person-centred care. Despite this, there continue to be deficits in care (see, for example, MENCAP, 2007).

In contrast, Ming-Li's approach to the older Chinese research participants suggests recognition and appraisal respect, the latter bestowed on the basis of their seniority. Although, as Middleton suggests, self-respect is not dependent on the actions of others, the actions of others can diminish or enhance self-respect. In Debbie's case it is evident also how categorisation as a member of a stigmatised group (drug users) can lead to disrespectful responses from a teacher and a lack of respect for her as an individual and a mother. Whereas, the subsequent change in the way she was treated by the school staff following Debbie's intervention may have led to enhanced self-respect. Having previously excluded her from involvement in Jimmy's education, the teachers begin to acknowledge her and involve her in a way that suggests she is valued as an individual and as Jimmy's mother. Ming-Li's sensitivity to the older people and her awareness that she needs to negotiate suggest the importance of appreciating that research interviews have the potential to cause distress to participants.

But what follows from this? We may have more clarity regarding the range of objects of respect, types of respect and the relationship between respect and self-respect but we have not as yet outlined what respectfulness requires of the professional.

Stages of respect

Raz (2001), a philosopher of law, develops a theory of respect. Raz outlines a rather complex argument with a view to reconciling the universal nature of value with its dependence on social contexts and with human partiality. There are, according to Raz, paradigmatic universal values such as 'life, respect for people, and personal well-being' (Raz, 2001, p. 8). Raz describes 'the duty of respect for people' as a universal duty which arises from the intrinsic value of people, that is, that they are of value in themselves.

Raz is not a virtue theorist and builds rather on the deontology or duty-based approach of Kant that focuses on respect for the moral law and on treating people as ends in themselves rather than merely as means to an end. People are to be treated, therefore, in accord with their intrinsic value and not 'merely' for their instrumental value, for example, for their contribution or services to others.

Raz outlines different ways of relating to what is considered valuable (this might be people, literature, life or art). We can respect it or go further by engaging with it. He writes:

We must respect what is valuable and it is wrong not to do so. We have reason to engage with what is valuable, and it is intelligible that we should do so. Sometimes it is foolish, rash, weak, defective in some other specific way, or even irrational to fail to engage with what is of greater value than available alternatives, or to engage with what is of lesser value. But it is not, generally speaking, wrong to do so.

(Raz, 2001, p. 6)

Raz argues that respect comprises two stages in relation to value: acknowledging value; and preserving and not destroying it. Engagement is another stage of the appropriate response to value that goes beyond respect and, as indicated above, is optional. These stages are helpful in suggesting how practitioners might be respectful in their practice. We suggest that it is helpful to consider four rather than three stages and that there are weaker and stronger versions of respect.

Respect as acknowledgement of value

First, the *acknowledgement of value*, the first stage suggested by Raz, (2001) means that our thoughts, imagining and emotions should be appropriate to the value of the object in question. Professional ethics and codes provide guidance on what the appropriate objects of respect are (rights, autonomy, individuality, dignity and so on) and the idea 'I acknowledge the value of each of these' seems legitimate. It is less clear what thoughts, imaginings and emotions are appropriate in relation to each of these objects when there is conflict, when effectively we need to prioritise one value-object over another. It seems we need also to strive to acknowledge value when we find it difficult, for example, when we work with service users we do not like or when we find the expression of their autonomy challenging. It seems plausible that the demonstration of good manners or politeness could serve as an acknowledgement of value. However, at best it could only be a beginning.

It is important to distinguish respect from politeness. Comte-Sponville (2002, p. 7) writes of politeness as 'the first virtue'. He says:

Politeness doesn't care about morality, and vice versa. If a Nazi is polite, does that change anything about Nazism or the horrors of Nazism? No. It changes nothing, and that nothing is the very hallmark of politeness. A virtue of pure form, of etiquette and ceremony! A show of virtue, its appearance and nothing more.

Comte-Sponville argues that politeness is a value, albeit an ambiguous one as 'it can clothe both the best and the worst, which makes it suspect'. He goes on to discuss politeness as the 'first virtue' in the sense that morality starts there. (Comte-Sponville (2002, p. 11) says of politeness:

> Politeness is only a beginning but at least it is that. To say 'please' or 'excuse me' is to pretend to be respectful; to say 'thank you' is to pretend to be grateful. And it is with this show of respect and this show of gratitude that both respect and gratitude begin. Just as nature imitates art, morality imitates politeness, which imitates morality.

If respectfulness is equated with a generalised politeness, its ethical foundations seem precarious. Politeness is something that can as easily be put in the service of what is solely self-serving rather than of something that demonstrates concern for or love of others. Returning to the situations of Debbie and Ming-Li there may have been differences in their views of the adequacy of acknowledgement in comprising respect. In Debbie's situation, acknowledgement would not have gone far enough and more active respect-promoting interventions were required. Ming-Li's story reveals a lack of respectfulness in terms of the lack of acknowledgement of people with learning disabilities (in the 1960s institution) whereas the older Chinese research participants are treated quite differently.

Respect as preservation and non-destruction

Raz outlines the second stage of respect as *preservation and non-destruction*. There is, according to Raz (2001, p. 162), 'a general reason to preserve what is of value'. Raz (p. 161) gives the example of respect in relation to the work of Michelangelo:

> Respect for Michelangelo's work consists primarily in acknowledging his achievement in what we say, and think, and in caring for the preservation of the work. This fact reflects another: one need not be among those who spend time examining it and admiring it. Not everyone need be an art connoisseur, or a devotee of Michelangelo's work. But everyone ought to respect his work.

Respecting the work of Michelangelo, then, requires acknowledgement of its value, non-destruction and, according to Raz, caring for its preservation. Preservation and non-destruction in relation to autonomy, dignity or people more generally has rather different implications to preservation and non-destruction in relation to art. Non-destruction in the example of art is achieved by, for example, not scratching, burning or pouring coffee over it. In the case of human relationships non-destruction is likely to be more subtle and nuanced and indeed the idea of destruction may appear too extreme. We could, for example, opt for not harming or not wronging and these are legitimate ethical rules. However, holding with the language of non-destruction reminds us, most acutely, of human vulnerability and fallibility. Humans have, for example, the potential to enhance and diminish the dignity of others.

We suggest that it might be more helpful to regard non-destruction as the second stage and preservation the third stage of respect and not, as Raz suggests, one stage. If, for example, Debbie had remained silent in the meeting with Jimmy's teachers, she personally would not have been destructive towards Lorraine, Jimmy's mother. More was, however, required to further her cause, to demonstrate respect for Lorraine. Debbie needed to be more active and to preserve Lorraine's dignity in the face of prejudice and exclusion. Ming-Li appears aware of the potential for harm or distress in the research interviews and talks of negotiating consent with the older Chinese participants as she moves to new and potentially challenging topics.

Respect and engagement

Engagement is the next stage – our fourth stage – and, Raz suggests, goes beyond respect. He writes of engaging with value in 'appropriate ways'. It is acknowledgement, preservation and non-destruction that he takes to relate to respect but these are 'not enough for a fulfilled life' (p. 163). Respect in relation to the health and social care professions requires more than this. It requires also engagement. A comment by Raz (2001, p. 148) suggests that his view of engagement is compatible with an Aristotelian approach to virtue ethics:

> Engaging with intrinsic goods in the right way and with the right spirit (and both way and spirit differ for a tennis match and for Proust) is good for one in and of itself, in one of many possible ways.

Although we may quibble as to whether tennis counts as an intrinsic good, it seems plausible that the appropriate exercise of engagement, as part of respectfulness, needs to be considered in relation to particular circumstances and can contribute to individual flourishing. A weaker and stronger view of respect is then discernible. The weaker view comprises the first three stages of correct response to value, that is, in acknowledging and not destroying and preserving (or promoting) objects of value. A stronger view would include also engagement. Being respectful in professional practice would seem to include the stronger view. This is likely to contribute to the flourishing of practitioners and service users. In relation to engaging with value in 'appropriate ways', Raz (pp. 162–163) gives the examples of listening to music, reading novels and rock climbing:

> Ultimately, value is realised when it is engaged with. There is a sense in which music is there to be appreciated in listening and playing, novels to be read with understanding, friendships to be pursued, dances to be joined in, and so on. Merely thinking of valuable objects and preserving them is a mere preliminary to engaging with value [...] Yet, obviously no one has to engage with all valuable objects. We need not read all the novels, listen to all the music, climb all the mountains, go to all the parties, dance in all the dances, which are worthwhile.

Similarly it may be argued that practitioners need not engage with all objects of value and it is sufficient that they acknowledge, do not destroy them and preserve them. This might be said, for example, of work environments or the car park attendant as objects of respect. When, however, we discuss respect in relation to service users and their families or colleagues, engagement is what is required. How practitioners engage with such objects of value in 'appropriate ways' requires consideration.

The significance of engagement in professional practice is not a new idea. Thurgood (2004, p. 650) writes of engagement in mental health nursing as follows:

> Establishing and maintaining relationships with clients that are experienced as helpful is fundamental to engagement. To do this requires nurses to learn about their clients' unique perspectives and to respect them as valid and meaningful. Respect for the client's

viewpoint provides the basis for collaborative working and open negotiation around informed choices for care and treatment.

Engagement as the final stage of respect goes beyond acknowledgment, non-destruction and preservation and requires the use of the self in developing relationships and getting to know and understand the perspective of those people with whom practitioners work. It also suggests the need for optimism, tenacity, compassion, professional wisdom and an aspiration to flourishing on the part of the practitioner.

All four stages of respect – acknowledgement, non-destruction, preservation and engagement – are necessary components of a meaningful and professional approach to respecting people and being a respectful practitioner. So how do these stages relate to the examples of Debbie and Ming-Li? That Debbie acknowledges the value of Lorraine and Billy as worthwhile human beings appears evident in her narrative. Her account suggests that the stages are not necessarily sequential but, rather, run together. Debbie's sensitivity to Lorraine's problems and her work with her suggest that she is acknowledging, not destroying, preserving and engaging. Debbie's knowledge of Lorraine and her commitment to respecting and helping her result in her challenging the prejudices of teachers and bringing about some positive changes, thus promoting non-discriminatory practice and social inclusion. Debbie's description of the teacher's response as 'disgusting' suggests an emotional reaction. Nussbaum (2004) describes disgust as a 'powerful emotion' generally associated with responses to repulsive substances and rotting matter but also with a social dimension. A connection might be made between disgust and fear or hatred of groups or individuals. Nussbaum (2004, p. 99) suggests that the 'core idea' of disgust is that the self might be contaminated and says that 'emotion expresses a possible contaminant'.

In sharing her experiences of working in an institution in the 1960s, Ming-Li describes practices that were dehumanising. Elsewhere in her interview she gives examples of efforts she made to improve care but it seems that the value or dignity (Gallagher, 2004) of people with learning disabilities was not acknowledged and their humanity is not preserved. Ming-Li's narrative also suggests that there was no meaningful engagement between practitioners and service users. Respectfulness was, therefore, not present in either a weak or a strong sense. In contrast, Ming's Li's work with the older Chinese research participants suggests respectfulness in both senses.

We have suggested, building on the work of Raz, four stages of respect: acknowledgement, non-destruction, preservation and active engagement. These stages appear also to support the development of self-respect in oneself as a professional and in service users.

The virtue of respectfulness

We have suggested that truly engaging with people, the fourth stage of respect, entails an aspiration to flourishing and professional activity that requires appropriate dispositions. Practitioners can act respectfully and can 'do' respect by acknowledging value, not destroying and preserving the dignity and autonomy of those they work with. Such actions suggest the virtue of respectfulness, however as with other virtues, they may not represent composite or global respectfulness. It is possible to be disposed to, for example, acknowledge and not destroy but refrain from preserving or engaging with objects of respect. It is also possible to be respectful in some but not all domains, for example, to be respectful to service users and families in a work setting but not to students or to some groups of people outside work. It is useful to think in terms of there being 'modules' of respectfulness.

As with other virtues, there are corresponding vices. The doctrine of the mean, explained in Chapter 3, entails considering virtues in relation to excess or deficiency. The deficiency, mean and excess in relation to respectfulness and self-respectfulness appear to be somewhat different. The virtue or mean of respectfulness, for example, suggests vices in the form of an excess as deference or sycophancy, and the deficiency as being disrespectful. The virtue or mean of self-respectfulness suggests vices in the form of a deficiency as servility and an excess as arrogance or grandiosity.

A demonstration of respectfulness requires the exercise of professional wisdom. The two vignettes suggest how nuanced and challenging practice situations can be and how, at times, it is not easy to know what is the most respectful thing to do. If Debbie had deferred to the teacher and accepted her view, it is plausible that she may be considered to have the vice of deference or servility. If Ming-Li had been arrogant and made assumptions regarding consent, she is unlikely to have been respectful. As discussed earlier, self-respectfulness is predominantly a self-regarding virtue, although arguably it is a necessary component of respectfulness and respectfulness is predominantly other-regarding. It is other-regarding in that it is directed towards other people, including service users, and will generally contribute towards their overall flourishing.

In relation to Debbie's situation, we cannot say with any certainty that she demonstrated composite or global respectfulness or modules of respectfulness. This is not possible given the limited data we have and the fact that this is but one vignette. Debbie's account does suggest, however, that she was 'being for the good' and that her work was undertaken within a framework of core values that she felt underpinned social work and perhaps also were directed towards a service ideal. Similarly, Ming-Li's work with Chinese older people suggested sensitivity to, and respect for, culture and autonomy.

Strategies for practice and professional education

In addition to lectures and seminars exploring the philosophical underpinning of respect and respectfulness, four strategies seem particularly relevant to the promotion of respectfulness: role modelling; reflective practice; engaging with examples from literature and the media; and the use of drama.

Role modelling

One of the ways, it has been suggested, that we learn how to be virtuous is to observe and learn from people we consider particularly good or ideal professionals. They are, effectively, exemplars of virtue. In relation to the virtue of respectfulness, there are opportunities to learn from and engage with role models in the classroom, in practice and elsewhere. If educators treat students with respect and approach them respectfully and if professionals model respectfulness in their encounters with service users, families, students and other professionals, then students and novice professionals are exposed to this and there is the potential to learn and to develop.

Health and social care professionals who assume roles in the public or political sphere have, arguably, a particular responsibility to ensure that their demeanour is supportive of the service ideal and upholds the reputation of the profession.

Reflective practice

Professionals (and people generally) are subject to limitations of rationality, sympathy and resources. They are, in short, fallible with the potential to thwart the flourishing of others resulting in harm and distress. This is particularly relevant in relation to the virtue of respectfulness. Disrespectfulness towards service users is well documented, pointing to ethical failings on the part of individuals and institutions. Reflective practice is a significant strategy in helping professionals to become more aware of their limitations and potential to promote human flourishing.

Blackburn (1999) argues that reflection is important in the way reading novels or listening to music is good, in itself and for its own sake. Reflection enables professionals (and others) to consider what they do, how to be and to evaluate their own perspectives in relation to others and to engage in self-scrutiny. This appears then also to encompass reflection on practice and on self. In relation to respectfulness, the key areas for reflection would include the following: How does my perspective on respect and respectfulness compare with that of others? How do I 'do' respect in everyday professional practice? And how might I develop the virtue of respectfulness?

MacIntyre (1999, p. 71) writes of the importance of reflection in relation to moral development. He writes that we need to:

> make the transition from accepting what we are taught by those earliest teachers to making our own independent judgements about goods, judgements that we are able to justify rationally to ourselves and to others as furnishing us with good reasons for acting in this way rather than that.

In addition to the ability to stand back from and to be able to evaluate our desires, to engage effectively in self-scrutiny, MacIntyre (1999, p. 96) also points to the possibility of fallibility regarding self-reflection and highlights the importance of social relationships in affirming and correcting self-knowledge. MacIntyre (1999, p. 97) gives good reasons for the importance of friendship and collegiality but he also points to the possibility of fallibility whereby friends and colleagues may lack the virtues necessary to develop and sustain practical reasoning. It is, therefore, important that practitioners retain an independent mind so that they can engage in critical self-appraisal and conclude or act differently.

Engagement with the medical humanities

Fictional and biographical literature, film and theatre can also enhance our understanding of respect and respectfulness. One extract that illustrates well some of the challenges of being respectful in everyday care practice comes from Alan Bennett's book, *Untold Stories*.[3]

Bennett writes of the experience of visiting his mother in a nursing home in Weston-super-Mare, England. He finds that she is wearing a 'fluorescent-orange cardigan' and a skirt that she would, he surmises, have considered 'common'. Bennett poignantly describes how his efforts to get a response from his mother are in vain. Mrs Bennett's carers, on the other hand, take a different approach. Bennett (2005, pp. 117–119) writes:

> And so it seems with Mam, as nothing I ever say provokes a response: no smile; no turn of the head even.
>
> The staff do it differently; make a good deal more noise than I do for a start, and one of the maids now erupts into the room and seizes Mam's hand, stroking her face and kissing her lavishly.
>
> 'Isn't she a love!
>
> 'Aren't you a love!
>
> 'Aren't we pretty this morning!
>
> 'Who's going to give me a kiss?'
>
> The dialogue makes me wince and the delivery of it seems so much bad acting better directed at a parrot or a Pekinese. But, irritatingly, Mam seems to enjoy it, this grotesque performance eliciting far more of a response than is achieved by my less condescending and altogether more tasteful contribution.
>
> Mam's face twitches into a parody of a smile, her mouth opens in what she must think is a laugh and she waves her hand feebly in appreciation, all going to show, in my view, that taste and discrimination has gone along with everything else [...]
>
> 'Aren't you good, Lily? You've eaten all your mince.'
>
> And Mam purses her lips over her toothless gums for a rewarding kiss. Twenty years ago she would have been as embarrassed by this affectation of affection as I am. But that person is dead or forgotten anyway, living only in the memory of this morose

---

[3] This example was used in Gallagher, A. (2007) 'The respectful nurse', *Nursing Ethics*, vol. 14, no. 3, pp. 360–371.

middle-aged man who turns up every fortnight, if she's lucky, and sits there expecting his affection to be deduced from the way he occasionally takes her hand, stroking the almost transparent skin before putting it sensitively to his lips.

No. Now she is Lily who has eaten all her mince and polished off her Arctic Roll, and her eyes close, her mouth opens and her head falls sideways on the pillow.

'She's a real card is Lily. We always have a laugh.'

'Her name's actually Lilian', I say primly.

'I know, but we call her Lily'.

Bennett is in a position to know about and to inform the reader about his mother's past preferences and preferred name. He acknowledges that his efforts to engage with his mother are unsuccessful and that the noisy and affectionate interventions of the staff get a response. In relation to respectfulness we might ask: What types of respect are suggested in this example in relation to actions of the staff? What stages of respect are evident? Were the responses of Mrs Bennett's carers respectful? In what ways? How might their responses have been more respectful?

Use of drama

Langen (2003) discusses the potential of drama in enabling students to learn about 'respect for persons'. He uses a particular system designed for groups called *Themenzentriertes Theater* (TZT or theme-centred theatre). Although Langen describes how this might be used in relation to a particular perspective on respect, drawn from the ethical theory of Immanuel Kant, it is equally relevant to developing respectfulness as a virtue. There are various stages of this technique. The introductory phase has three exercises. First, the entrance exercise invites students to show respect to peers by offering a greeting or a salute; the second exercise requires students to move around the room without any contact; the third exercise involves the students being split into two groups (nobles and servants). The servants have to demonstrate respect to the nobles and then the students reverse roles. The second phase involves the formation of small groups. The exercises invite students to consider differences, such as height, in relation to respect and to consider what categories of people deserve respect. The third phase involves consideration of a situation or scenario and the students' experience of how they might show and receive respect from the positions of people who are powerful and those who are powerless. The fourth phase, realisation, focuses on the kind of situations service users might experience (for example, in not getting and getting respect). Phase five involves improvisation where students are invited to work together with a view to creating a sculpture titled 'respect'. The final exit phase provides the opportunity for students to express what they had gained from the TZT process. Langen (2003, p. 122) explains the potential benefits of TZT as follows:

> teaching ethical theories through the use of TZT could become a chance to change abstract and marginalised knowledge into useful skills integrated into professional action.

It seems possible also that TZT has the potential to enable students to consider the meaning of 'being respectful' and to learn from the example of others.

Concluding comments

There is much rhetoric relating to respect in contemporary professional ethics literature. There is also much good practice and positive innovations that promote respectful, person- and family-centred approaches to care. Research and media reports, however, suggest that the experiences of service users within health and social care are not as good as they could be. Practitioners and institutions are not always respectful of their dignity, autonomy and individuality. Ming-Li's account of dehumanised and disrespectful care in an institution in the 1960s is not, sadly, unique nor confined to history. There is, therefore, no room for complacency.

Much of the discussion of respect and respectfulness in this chapter has been influenced by the work of Raz, who is not a virtue theorist but rather situates his work in a deontological or duty-based theory. The stages of respect that include engagement provide a helpful framework on which to think about and operationalise respectfulness in everyday practice. That is not to say, however, that this is always straightforward. Practice is complex, challenging and, at times, ambiguous. The vignettes suggest the importance of respectfulness for a social worker and a nurse researcher. Debbie's reference to 'basic respect' lends support to her disposition and actions to advocate for the rights and interests of a woman who had, effectively, been excluded by other professionals. Her account suggests also the significance of other virtues, for example, courage and practical wisdom.

Ming-Li's account introduces some different and, in some ways, more challenging conceptual questions regarding the relationship between respectfulness and different cultures. Ming-Li came from a traditional Chinese culture, was socialised into cultural norms that emphasise respect for seniority, experienced what she considers to be disrespectful cultures of care and is now engaged in research where she talks of the need for sensitivity to the cultural biographies of participants. Respectfulness needs, therefore, to be contextualised or situated within particular cultures. Professionals and others need to understand how ethical failings within some institutional cultures might be avoided and how other institutional cultures might be supported to promote flourishing.

Chapter 7

Trustworthiness

Introduction

On traditional accounts of professionalism, trust, it is claimed, lies at the heart of the relationship between professionals and the users of services. This entails that service users believe or assume that professionals are competent to perform their defined job roles and will not deliberately let them down or harm them (an attitude on the part of service users); and that professionals are, in fact, committed to and competent in performing their specified roles well (a disposition to feel, think and behave in a certain kind of way on the part of professionals).

The paradigm relationship of trust in a professional context is one where the service users are trusting and the professionals are trustworthy. This is an asymmetrical, one-way relationship, with the service user as trustor and the professional as trustee. Although in some contexts the relationship is reciprocal or two-way (the professional is also trusting towards the service user and the service user is trustworthy), in professional work the important direction of the relationship is that the service user can (potentially) trust the professional. In health and social care work, in particular, there may be many occasions when professionals do not trust patients or service users to follow their advice or instructions, to look after themselves competently or even to be committed to behaving in ways that the professionals judge to be in the service users' own best interests. Indeed, the service users' limited competence, or lack of commitment to caring for themselves properly, may be the very reason why they seek (or are referred for) professional help in the first place.

This feature of people using professional services (that they may lack the expertise, competence, motivation or legal authority to perform certain tasks themselves) means that sometimes they are not able to assess the competence or commitment of the professionals working with them. This also makes them particularly vulnerable to exploitation or abuse. In some cases, especially in social work, a service user may be in an involuntary relationship with a professional and would be unwilling to trust the professional to understand and support their self-defined interests. So what is left at the heart of the professional relationship in cases such as these is the trustworthiness of the professional to perform a defined and socially sanctioned role, regardless of whether the actual service users are able or willing to place trust. Not surprisingly, therefore, several texts on professional ethics include trustworthiness as one of the key virtues of the practitioner, for example, Beauchamp and Childress (2001, p. 82) and Oakley and Cocking (2001), although in neither of these texts is there an extended analysis of professional trustworthiness.

This chapter will explore what it means for a professional to be regarded as 'trustworthy' and how this is accomplished and sustained as a professional virtue. In order to do this we will first explore the nature of trust. We will also consider the claim that there is currently a climate of mistrust of professionals, which both engenders and is engendered by increasing regulation and control of their behaviour, considering the implications of this for the idea that the trustworthiness of professionals is at the heart of professional work.

Vignettes

The vignettes that follow offer accounts relevant to trustworthiness from two different perspectives: that of the professional and that of the service user. The first vignette is based on material from an interview with a nurse conducted for this book, while the second draws on an interview with a service user presented in Cree and Davis (2007, p. 114).

1) The importance of trustworthiness in the paediatric nurse

Lynne is a very experienced paediatric nurse. When asked to talk about ethical qualities relevant to professional practice, trustworthiness was one of the qualities she emphasised:

I think trust is very important as well, because, especially with children, *the parents need to trust you*, you know, they've brought their sick child into hospital and they're handing it over to strangers. OK, you wear a uniform, you're qualified, but you're still a stranger to them; and you've got someone who is very, very important to them and *they expect you to able to care for the child …* Probably a lot of stuff written in the press has made people question, you know maybe years ago when they walked onto the ward and they see a nurse or a doctor, there was this respect, and *a presumption that the person was trustworthy*. But nowadays we know from what's written in the press that things are not always that way.

I think as a nurse *you have to work quite hard to build a trusting relationship* so that maybe they can leave their child on the ward to go home and do things, or bring clothes in for the child or go and get themselves a cup of tea; and they're not going to do that until they feel you are not going to harm their child and that you also know what you are doing. So I think as a nurse you have to work quite quickly to get that, *build up the sort of trust*, you know, to *come across as competent but not being sort of threatening* and someone who is quite likeable nowadays not too set in their ways, a bit flexible.

When asked for a specific example, Lynne gave the following account:

Well I can remember I went to do a shift on a ward that I had been working on but I had left and I came back, so I was the bank nurse. There was a small baby that had quite a serious heart defect so I went in and introduced myself and made a quick assessment of the child and his mother was there and she looked very anxious and she asked me what I knew. Or she said something to me about her child and I didn't say very much and she said: 'You do know what's wrong with him, don't you?' I didn't know how much she knew so I sort of said basically what I knew: that he had quite a serious hole in his heart and that seemed to satisfy her. And then, but she stayed in the room and I did a few other bits and pieces and eventually she left the room and it really struck me *the importance of building up a trusting relationship between the parent and the nurse*. She didn't know me, she hadn't seen me on the ward before so I was this strange person who had walked in and

she was worried about her baby and I could see at the beginning that she probably felt that she couldn't refuse to have me looking after her child but she wanted to suss me out and see what I was capable of. And the child had been in hospital for quite a long time, she had a good idea about what people did when they came in, first of all, to see a child and how the equipment worked and the sort of thing, the checks that people made. And I very much got the opinion that she was trying to work out whether I was competent or not and I had this feeling of having to try and prove myself to her. But then once we worked through that she was fine and it was a very good shift in the end.
(Source: interview. Our italics)

2) Helena's experience of a social worker

Helena was diagnosed as 'learning disabled' when she was 11, as she was 'slow at learning to read and write'. She then attended a special school until she was 18 years old, which, in her view, 'offered no education at all'. According to Helena, she learnt to read and write at the age of 13 with the help of her sister. Yet when she left school the headmaster indicated that she could not go to work because she was not able to read and write. Two years later she had tried two work scheme placements, which she found boring. One day she announced at the end of a day centre session she was attending that she was no longer prepared to stay on training schemes. This prompted the day centre to arrange for a visit to Helena and her family from a social worker, Alison, who worked for a local disability employment scheme. Helena commented about Alison:

> She was the first one who was interested in us. We sat down and had a talk about my future and work and we told her what we wanted and what I would like to do […] I felt good because it gave me confidence that someone wanted to know what I wanted to do.

Alison supported Helena in looking for work, and Helena eventually found a job placement as a part-time administrative assistant in a university. Helena was surprised that Alison did not disappear from the scene at this point, commenting that:

> she stopped on. She said it was because she had to sort out my benefits when I went to work […] *she really knew what she was*

doing. I trusted her. She has always given me the right advice [...] she *always* had time to sit and talk. She was very good at explaining. If I didn't know something I could *always* ask her a question and she would *always* answer you.

After three years, Alison suggested that Helena should inquire about a full-time permanent job at the university. Although Helena was surprised at this suggestion, she trusted Alison, followed her advice, was successful, and six years later at the time of the interview was still working as a university administrator. Helena has kept contact with Alison, commenting:

I last saw her about three months ago to help me fill in a benefit form. She still helps me. *It feels good knowing she is there for me.*
(Source: Modified from Cree and Davis, 2007, pp. 107, 113–114. Our italics)

Reflections

The first vignette is written from the perspective of the professional (a paediatric nurse) in whom other people (particularly parents of children in the hospital where she works) 'need to trust'. The characterisation of this type of situation (parents handing over the care of sick children to nurses) as one where trust is an issue has been made by the nurse, Lynne. She has observed from experience how important it is for parents to feel that the nurses caring for their children are not going to harm them and that they are competent at their jobs. She reports how hard she has to work to build a trusting relationship. Her particular example of coming onto a ward as a 'bank nurse' exemplifies the point made in her general discussion about parents having to trust 'strangers'. The mother is already well-versed in the way the ward works and how the nurses behave. So when Lynne comes in as a 'bank nurse' (a temporary role that by its very nature is a disembedded and replaceable one), despite the fact that she is qualified and wears a uniform (signs of commitment and competence), the mother is immediately suspicious. Lynne feels she has to 'prove' herself quite quickly. She describes how to do this in her earlier discussion of situations like this. The nurse has to 'come across' as a certain kind of person (competent, not threatening and flexible).

Lynne only uses the term 'trustworthy' once to refer to the kind of person a nurse is/should be. From what Lynne says, it is clear that she believes herself to be trustworthy. Although she does not explicitly describe the details of her nursing experience in the extract quoted here, we know she is very experienced. So we get the impression of someone who is committed to caring well for young children and who is competent in her practice. But she has to communicate her commitment and competence to the parents of the children in her care. Lynne talks generally about having to 'work' to 'build up' trust. What is important in the case of the particular mother and child that Lynne gives as an example is Lynne's performance as a nurse who can be trusted in this situation.

The second vignette, written from the perspective of a service user (Helena), gives an account of how a social worker (Alison) has given her long-term support and advice. Helena says she trusts Alison, by implication because 'she really knew what she was doing' (Alison is competent, perhaps even 'expert' in her field) and 'she has *always* given me the right advice' (she has a good track record). Somewhat to Helena's surprise, Alison has maintained contact over a period of years and still gives help. Alison's commitment means Helena feels that she knows 'she is there for me'. In this vignette, the social worker has shown herself to be trustworthy over a long period and Helena is giving an account of a long-standing relationship. This is a very different kind of situation to that depicted in the first vignette, about the relationship between a nurse and the patients/families she is caring for. In the hospital situation, nurses come and go, and patients may only stay for short periods of time. So in order to gain trust, the nurse has to perform very quickly according to the pre-existing role expectations parents have of a paediatric nurse. In the second vignette, on the other hand, the service user has few expectations of the social worker, so the slow discovery that she can be relied upon to give support and good advice is surprising and greatly appreciated.

Trust

The two vignettes focus more on service users' attitudes of trust towards professionals than on the trustworthiness of the professionals *per se*. However, as noted in the introduction, the trustworthiness of the professionals is part of the relationship of trust, along with the trusting attitude of the service users. Like 'care', we could say that 'trustworthiness' is a relational virtue in that the concept of one person being trustworthy is based on an assumption of others (justifiably) trusting that person. So before examining what it means to be trustworthy, we will first explore the nature of trust.

In everyday speech, in addition to talking about placing trust in people ('I trust the nurse not to harm my baby'), we often talk about trusting objects, systems or institutions ('I trust the hospital computer system to keep track of patient records'). Clearly in this chapter, we are interested in trust between people rather than the trustworthiness of computer systems. However, the difference between interpersonal trust and other uses of the term 'trust' highlights some important distinctions that have been made in the literature between different types of trust, or, what should strictly speaking be regarded as 'trust', and what could be characterised as 'confidence' or 'faith'. In expressing 'trust' in the hospital computer system, we could be said to be expressing a belief in its reliability – that it will do the job it is designed to do, that there are systems in place to check for inaccuracies, that the staff operating the system are well-qualified and trained, that appropriate security is in place if records are to be sent elsewhere and so on. This is about predictability and reliability, whereas trust in people is, as Seligman (1997, p. 17) puts it, 'tied to some psychological orientation'. Seligman, along with other sociologists such as Giddens (1990) and Luhmann (1979, 1988), prefers to use the term 'confidence' rather than 'trust' to refer to institutions or systems, to differentiate it from trust in people that is 'built upon mutuality of response and involvement' (Giddens, 1990, p. 114).

While reliability does seem to be part of interpersonal trust, there is more to trust between people than just reliability. Taking the second vignette, Helena's trust in her social worker, Alison, is certainly based upon Helena's assessment from past experience of Alison's reliability, which leads Helena to expect that Alison will be there for her when needed. In the second quotation from Helena when she says of Alison, 'I trusted her', she describes how Alison 'stopped on' (that is, continued to support her) and uses the word 'always' four times when describing Alison's behaviour. But is there not something more to Helena's attitude of trust than simply Alison's reliability? Some philosophers have argued that if we trust someone, we not only expect that they will behave reliably (according to their earlier promises, or accepted standards of a role such as 'social worker'), but that they have a certain kind of motive towards us. For Baier (1986), this is a motive of good will. Although Helena does not describe her views of Alison's motivation in any detail, she does say Alison 'was interested in us' and 'wanted to know what I wanted to do'. We could imagine interviewing Alison about her motives and her giving a response suggesting a general interest in Helena's progress and a desire to give her as much support as possible. This would be consistent with Alison having a 'motive of good will' towards Helena.

However, while a motivation of good will in the trustee may be a feature of many trusting relationships, is it a necessary feature of all trusting relationships? What if, when questioned further, Alison said, 'I am using my work with Helena as a case study for my professional doctorate. I need to develop a good relationship with her so I can sustain the work over several years'? Does this mean that we would then judge Alison to be reliable but not trustworthy in this situation? It would probably depend upon whether Alison gave the impression of being genuinely interested in Helena, whereas really she was not. But how do we tell the difference between a genuine interest and a 'fake' or 'instrumental' interest? In a professional relationship the role requires professionals to treat the people they are working with in certain kinds of ways. In the case of a disability employment social worker, getting to know the service user, showing an interest in them and building their confidence in themselves are all part of what it takes to do the job well. So the motivation we might expect in a professional social worker or nurse is the motivation to do the job well. Nevertheless, when there is a long-standing relationship between a professional and service user, we probably do also expect a strong motive of 'good will' towards service users to pertain. Walker (2006, p. 82) suggests these relationships involve mixed forms of trust:

> We expect them [professionals] to be competent and to be motivated by recognition and commitment to fulfilling their professional or occupational responsibilities, but we also think – or want to think – that they have personal concern and regard for us and will be moved by it.

Govier (1997) gives an account of trust, which entails the trustor having expectations of benign behaviour based on beliefs about the other person's motivation and competence. This may be a less onerous burden on the trustee than 'good will' in a professional context. Govier (1997, p. 6) gives an account of trust as a complex attitude on the part of the trustor involving four features, which can be summarised as follows:

1. Expectations of benign behaviour based on beliefs about a person's motivation and competence;

2. An attribution of general integrity by the trustor to the person trusted;

3. An acceptance by the trustor of risk and vulnerability;

4. A disposition on the part of the trustor to interpret the trusted person's actions favourably.

This outline of the features of trust probably fits many of the situations encountered in professional life. It would certainly seem to fit Helena's account of her trust in Alison. She clearly expects Alison to give good advice and to act benignly towards her. The fact that Alison is described as 'being there for' Helena implies a kind of integrity. While Helena does not stress her own vulnerability, this is implied in her description of her situation prior to meeting Alison as one in which she has been subject to treatment based on the assumption that she has limited abilities. She is clearly at the time of speaking disposed to interpret Alison's behaviour favourably.

As a characterisation of trust in general, however, the 'expectation of benign behaviour' may also be inadequate. Walker (2006, pp. 77–78) gives the example of engaging a hired killer to kill someone, and trusting the killer to commit the murder, which is not 'benign'. The expectation of benign behaviour, she claims, only fits cases where we trust people to do things at discretion that could harm our interests, or to behave quite generally in ways that do not harm or threaten anyone. In the professional context, the expectation of benign behaviour is quite common. However, it is possible to imagine cases where this does not pertain – for example, a situation in a care home where a social care worker repeatedly physically restrains a young woman when she exhibits violent behaviour towards other residents. The young woman does not expect benign behaviour from the worker, but we might say she trusts the worker to act in the ways expected of a care professional (that is, to use the permitted methods of restraint, not to torture and tease her and so on).

Walker (2006, p. 80) offers an alternative view of trust, which may fit this kind of situation better. For her, trust involves normative expectations of others – that they will behave in a certain sort of way; it involves regarding them as potentially responsible and responsive. She offers a generic account of interpersonal trust as:

> A kind of reliance on others whom we expect (perhaps only implicitly or unreflectively) to behave as relied upon (e.g., in specified ways, in ways that fulfil an assumed standard, or in ways so as to achieve relied-upon outcomes) and to behave that way in the awareness (if only implicit or unreflective) that they are liable to be held responsible for failing to do so or make reasonable efforts to do so.

This characterisation of trust leaves motivation open, and takes account of the fact that people may be moved in many ways to do what they know they are responsible for doing. As Walker (2006, pp. 81–82) claims, it also enables us to regard some instances of trusting as dominated by cognitive assessments of reliability and others as more affective, based on optimistic or hopeful attitudes. What she calls 'hopeful trust' may be held when the outcomes we seek are not very likely. Or we may give trust hopefully to some people, in the anticipation that this may activate their sense of responsibility. This links with the idea of 'therapeutic trust' whereby, for example, a parent may trust a child to look after the cat, with the aim of developing the child's trustworthiness (Horsburgh, 1960; McLeod, 2006, p. 8).

If we accept Walker's account of trust as reliability with responsibility, then we might modify Govier's account of trust to replace the expectation of benign behaviour with two statements about reliability and responsibility. Trust would then entail the following:

1. Expectations that the person trusted will behave as relied upon;

2. Expectations that the person trusted will regard themselves as responsible for behaving in this way;

3. An attribution of general integrity by the trustor to the person trusted;

4. An acceptance by the trustor of risk and vulnerability;

5. A disposition on the part of the trustor to interpret the trusted person's actions favourably.

Trustworthiness

If this is what counts as 'trust', let us now consider the nature of 'trustworthiness'. At first we may be tempted to suppose that a trustworthy person is simply someone in whom others place their trust. However, we need to take account of situations where people mistakenly place trust. For example, we may trust someone to do something that is not within their competence or the remit of their role, while they are unaware of being trusted and have no feeling of responsibility for whatever is expected of them. It is important to include awareness of responsibility (even if this is implicit) in an account of trustworthiness. Hence we might describe a trustworthy person as someone who behaves as relied upon and is aware that they are liable to be held responsible for this behaviour.

In addition to unwanted trust, we also need to take account of the fact that it is possible for many people to place trust in someone who is, in fact, untrustworthy. To be trust*worthy* is more than simply being trust*able* (where the latter involves having the capacity to make/encourage people to trust). It is about being worthy of that trust. For example, many people trusted Harold Shipman, a British doctor who was convicted of systematically killing over 200 of his patients over a number of years (Carter and Ward, 2002; see also The Shipman Inquiry website for the reports). The relatives of the people who died gave accounts afterwards of how they trusted him to care for their families and perform the duties expected of a doctor. The trust was based partly on the fact that he was a doctor and inherent in that role is that its incumbent is trustworthy, but also because he developed relationships with his patients and their families that demonstrated (or appeared to demonstrate, we might say with hindsight) a commitment to their health and well-being. We might say, 'he appeared trustworthy'; or 'he was a trustable sort of chap', but not, with hindsight, that 'he was trustworthy'. People can (wrongly) place trust in people in a professional or personal role (like a doctor or an intimate partner) who turn out to be untrustworthy. This may be because either, like Shipman, they have been systematically and deliberately deceiving people all along or a person who has hitherto acted in ways consistent with being regarded as trustworthy, unexpectedly betrays the trust (such as the loyal partner of many years who suddenly engages in an extra-marital affair).

So although the concept of trustworthiness is intimately connected with placing trust, it may be the case that people mistakenly place trust in an untrustworthy person, or, indeed, fail to trust someone who is, in fact, trustworthy. The paradigm case of the latter is the prophetess Cassandra, daughter of Priam, King of Troy, whose predictions always turned out to be true, but whom nobody trusted as a prophetess. We might imagine that the doctor who succeeded Harold Shipman might have found some of Shipman's former patients initially reluctant to place their trust.

All sorts of reasons may influence whether people place their trust, including whether the person they are considering trusting can plausibly present herself as trustworthy, people's previous experience of being let down by others in similar situations, an assessment of how serious the consequences would be of being let down, the climate of trust in society generally and in the organisational/institutional setting of which the potentially trusting relationship is part.

Lynne, the paediatric nurse, had to do a lot of work to build a trusting relationship with the mother in the first vignette. She had to behave in a 'trustable' way. This would be partly because of what was at stake for the mother if Lynne let her down (the baby might die). But it may also be partly because the mother has heard about nurses who are untrustworthy – who make mistakes or who deliberately harm babies. In her account, Lynne alludes to this when she mentions the media in her initial remarks about developing trusting relationships in general in her role as a nurse. She refers to the past, when people would much more easily and quickly trust nurses, simply because they were nurses (wearing the uniform was enough). There was the assumption that professionals were trustworthy – they were committed to perform the role well and competent to do so. We might suggest this unquestioning trust would be a form of what O'Neill (2002) calls 'blind trust'. However, it is not quite the same as trusting a complete stranger in a non-professional context – for example, a passer-by in the street offering to hold a mother's baby while she looks for her purse. Built into the role of 'nurse' is the requirement to be trustworthy, and built into the hospital systems are procedures and programmes for vetting and educating nurses.

However, the point Lynne is making is that this is not enough for many people in the current climate of mistrust. For example, we might regard the mother in the first vignette as facing 'the Shipman problem'. Here is someone (Lynne) who looks the part (dressed in a nurse's uniform) but how does the mother know she is not a 'wolf in sheep's clothing'? For Lynne, on the other hand, this situation might be regarded as a weak version of 'the Cassandra problem'. Lynne is committed and competent (a trustworthy nurse) but she is not trusted initially. Unlike Cassandra, however, Lynne knows that if she proves herself, she will be trusted. She has to perform trustworthiness. It is just about possible to imagine a nurse who, like Cassandra, acts reliably according to the expectations of someone in her role and takes responsibility for her role (that is, she is trustworthy in the terms described above), yet is not trusted. However, this is an unusual type of situation. If it were not for the fact that Cassandra's plight was engineered by the Greek god Apollo, we might assume that she just did not know how to act the part (perhaps she looked shifty, spoke hesitantly or dressed oddly). In professional life, performance as a trustworthy person is important. This is not the whole of what counts as being trustworthy (as the Shipman case exemplifies), but if someone cannot perform as a trustworthy nurse or social worker, we might say they are not competent to fulfil their roles. For part of the professional role involves being able to make and maintain professional relationships, and if professionals do not come across as plausibly trustworthy, then this will be difficult. Whether we add this to our account of what it means to be trustworthy, or simply say it is another dimension of the professional role, is, perhaps, a matter of definition – of where we draw the boundaries between different virtues and competences. Arguably, however, we could add a third feature of trustworthiness to reliability and responsibility, namely, plausibility, or the ability to perform as trustworthy, which is particularly relevant to professionals, especially in the current climate. On this account, a trustworthy person is someone who:

- behaves as relied upon;
- is aware and accepts that they are liable to be held responsible for this behaviour;
- is able to give a plausible performance as a reliable and responsible person.

We will now consider the issue of declining public trust in professionals and its implications for conceptions of trustworthiness as at the heart of professional relationships.

Questioning the trustworthiness of professionals

Much has been written about the growing public mistrust of professionals. Well-publicised cases of professionals (like Shipman) deceiving or deliberately harming service users, or being incompetent or negligent in the performance of the tasks associated with their roles, are said to have reduced public trust in professionals in general (Banks, 2004; Chadwick & Levitt, 1997; O'Neill, 2002). This can be linked with changing societal attitudes and shifts in public policy more generally. A 'postmodernist' analysis would suggest that the specialisation of expertise and the growth of publicly available information in areas such as health and social care make it difficult for people to decide which source of information or advice is correct, best or most appropriate. So there is a much more questioning attitude towards 'experts'. Awareness and tolerance of risk is changing, with people seeking legal or contractual guarantees in relation to the process and outcomes of professional services. So there is much less reliance on personal relationships and more on institutionalised systems and structures.

As already noted, on traditional accounts of what it means to be a professional, trustworthiness is central. This view of professionalism, as grounded in an implicit or explicit oath whereby professionals commit themselves to serve humanity and do good rather than harm (Koehn, 1994), has trustworthiness built into its very nature. Since the people professionals are working with/for generally have less expertise or power in the area of life with which professionals are involved, these 'clients' or service users are vulnerable to deception or exploitation. So professional practitioners, in effect, give a promise not to take advantage of the people they are working with/ for; to use their power, knowledge and skills for good rather than ill, and generally to act in ways expected of people in their professional role. This version of professionalism, based on the notion of the individual practitioner committed to fulfilling their role as, for example, a 'good social worker', 'a good nurse' or a 'good doctor' (as someone who is both ethically good and practically competent), is epitomised in the Hippocratic oath, which until quite recently used to be sworn by doctors (Koehn, 1994, p. 60). Over time, some of these promises have been institutionalised into systems of professional recognition and control. So in assessing whether or how to engage with a professional service, users may also find themselves assessing their confidence in the systems and institutions of which the professionals are part. This might suggest that trustworthiness, which was once at the heart of the professional relationship, is either less important or irrelevant. This is one of the issues addressed by O'Neill (2002), who argued very eloquently in the BBC Reith Lectures that, in spite of all the rhetoric to the contrary, we do still place trust in professionals and all kinds of other people upon whose services and good will we rely.

Even if we espouse a 'thin'[1] version of professionalism, where professionals are bound by legal contracts and follow defined procedures and codes to complete many of their tasks, the people using their services will still find themselves needing to place trust in the individual professionals. First, while professionals are subject to increasing numbers of rules that prescribe how they should behave in particular circumstances, we do still have to trust them to follow the rules (assuming we believe the rules are good rules in the first place). Although there are systems of surveillance and reporting that attempt to ensure that the rules are followed, we know that these cannot be watertight. Secondly, even if we had complete confidence in all the rules and surveillance systems as developed, we still have to trust the people enforcing the rules and developing the systems. If we pursue this infinite regress of diminishing trust, then the impossibility of being able absolutely to guarantee a good and competent service becomes apparent, and as do the diminishing returns from investing in systems to regulate the regulators. Ironically, it could be argued, as more and more regulation and control is piled on in attempts to make professionals more 'trustworthy' (in the sense of reliable and plausible), the less motivated they are to be trustworthy (reliable and responsible).

So, whilst mistrust may be reported as being endemic and escalating, as O'Neill (2002) points out, we nevertheless do continue to place trust. For example, although I may say, 'I don't trust medical professionals', I nevertheless do continue to place my trust in at least some of them. If I decide to go ahead and have an appendectomy, I have to place my trust in the surgeon who is going to perform the operation. This fact may suggest a contradiction or inconsistency (I say one thing and do another) or a tendency to over-generalise (in stating that I believe that all medical professionals are untrustworthy

---

[1] By 'thin' we mean based on following procedures and contracts, rather than on the character traits and commitments of professional practitioners.

in all circumstances). Alternatively, or in addition, it may indicate slightly different senses of the term 'trust'. O'Neill tends to use the term 'placing trust' in these cases of trusting people to perform specific roles or tasks. So it might be the case that although in many respects I do not trust Ms Brown, the surgeon who is going to perform my operation (for example, I do not trust her to visit when she promised to explain the surgical procedures in detail), I do trust her to do a good job in performing the appendectomy. This suggests that it may be useful to distinguish between trusting someone fully (in all circumstances and in relation to all people) to behave in the expected way and trusting someone to do something specific (in particular circumstances and/or in relation to a particular set of people).

Let us now assume that Ms Brown is sick on the day of my operation and her assistant, Mr Green, replaces her. Mr Green looks relatively young and inexperienced, and although I do not completely trust Mr Green to do my operation well, I am forced to place my trust in him (in the sense of entrusting myself to his care) as I now have a burst appendix and he is the only surgeon available. This suggests a distinction between trusting someone wholeheartedly to do something, and trusting someone, but with reservations (or 'grudgingly'). We might want to say that if I only trust Mr Green grudgingly then I do not really trust him. Or perhaps 'grudging' trust is akin to 'hopeful trust' – the prediction for a good outcome may not be that great, but I have to take a risk. As we noted earlier, the essence of 'trust' is that it involves risk and there is no guarantee of a good outcome. If there were such a guarantee, then trust would be redundant. So we might want to characterise the current climate as one where both full and wholehearted trust (and certainly 'blind trust') are less easily created (by trustees) or given (by trustors). Hopeful, grudging and considered trust are more common. Grudging or pessimistic trust is most damaging to individuals, institutions and society. It is reinforced by a climate of regulation and surveillance and in turn tends to reinforce the need for more regulation. A professional who is grudgingly trusted may begin to behave in a grudgingly trustworthy way – going through the motions, exhibiting reliability without the motive of responsibility and plausibility.

This analysis suggests that it might be useful to think in terms of degrees of trust, from wholehearted to partial, as the following analysis suggests:

Wholehearted trust – this is a strong form of trust and may take a number of forms, for example:

▶ 'blind' – we place trust without questioning or even naively (for example, in the stranger who looks plausible).

▶ 'semi-blind' – we place trust based on role expectations (for example, trusting a nurse, even though she is unknown to us).

▶ 'considered' – we place trust based on experience, assessment or judgement (for example, Helena in the second vignette seems to trust Alison wholeheartedly based on her long experience of her).

Partial trust – we are not sure about either the person's commitment and/or their competence, so the trust we place may be

▶ hopeful/optimistic – we place trust hopefully in situations where we do not have much information to go on (this might be regarded as 'semi-blind'), but we hope the person will live up to our optimism.

▶ grudging/pessimistic – we reluctantly place trust, without much hope that the person will live up to our trust.

Does this mean there are also degrees of trustworthiness? If trustworthiness is a disposition to act reliably, plausibly and take responsibility for performance of roles and actions, then people can be regarded and may regard themselves as relatively reliable, relatively plausible and relatively responsible, depending on circumstances. In which case, it would make sense to also regard people as relatively trustworthy.

Potter (2002) makes the distinction, already referred to in Chapter 3, between 'specific trustworthiness' that is relative to particular relationships and 'full trustworthiness', which entails a disposition to be trustworthy towards everyone. It is the latter that she regards as the character trait that virtuous people possess. According to Potter (2002, p. 16), a trustworthy person (in the virtue sense of the term) is one who

> can be counted on, as a matter of the sort of person he or she is, to take care of those things that others entrust to one and (*following the Doctrine of the Mean*) whose ways of caring are neither excessive nor deficient.
>
> [emphasis in the original]

Those people who are fully trustworthy in this 'thick'[2] virtue sense would not only act in a trustworthy fashion in relation to all their professional roles and tasks, but also across their personal lives. This is a very strong claim, and it might be regarded more as an aspiration for most people, rather than a reality. Indeed, it is claims such as these, namely that virtues are enduring features of character that persist across all aspects of life, that have stimulated what has been called the 'situationist critique' of virtue ethics (as discussed in Chapter 3). This is a critique based particularly on the empirical results of a number of psychological experiments that show that the most significant factors influencing whether people act in ways that are, for example, kind, caring or trustworthy are variations in situations or circumstances, rather than people's motives or character (Doris, 2002; Harman, 1999).

However, trustworthiness as a virtue in professional life might be regarded as a form of specific trustworthiness, which nevertheless applies across all professional relationships and in all professional situations but not beyond these boundaries. This entails that we would expect Lynne (the nurse) and Alison (the social worker) to behave in a trustworthy fashion in all aspects of their professional lives, not just with mothers of small babies in a hospital ward or in one relationship with a particular service user, but also in clinics or case conferences and with colleagues, or members of the public encountered in the course of their work. We would expect, on a virtue ethics account of trustworthiness, that they would be motivated or committed to performing their professional roles competently and in accordance with the relevant professional values and service ideals about promoting health and social welfare.

The vignettes we have used, of course, only show Lynne and Alison performing in one type of situation with one type of patient or service user. These are cases that demonstrate a quite specific situational trustworthiness, which are indicative (but not proof) of a broader disposition towards trustworthy behaviour in the professional role. If we found that Lynne constantly promised the mother in the vignette that she would arrange to order a supply of special nappies (diapers) the next day, but she never did, we might regard her as untrustworthy in this respect, whilst still trusting her to

---

[2] By 'thick' we mean trustworthiness based on qualities of character rather than principles or contracts.

monitor the baby's heart condition, administer the required medication and generally care well for the baby's health. In which case we might say that Lynne is *relatively* trustworthy as a nurse, but we might not want to say she is trustworthy in the full virtue sense of the term. This reminds us that virtue is learned and developed with practice. We surely would not expect professionals to be perfect, but we do expect them to be as trustworthy as possible, particularly in important matters relating significantly to the health and well-being of service users and members of the public. When patients, service users or members of the public show their disappointment or suffering as a result of being let down, then professionals may be motivated to change their behaviour and, for example, develop a disposition to make fewer promises to service users or to keep even small promises (as in the hypothetical case of the special nappies).

Strategies for practice and professional education

Having explored at some length the nature of trustworthiness, we will now consider how this moral quality is developed and enhanced in professional practitioners.

Placing trust in trainee practitioners

We have already discussed the concept of 'hopeful' or 'optimistic' trust, whereby we place trust in people who may not yet be fully competent and have not yet had to take much responsibility. We do this in the anticipation that by being trusted, they will have an incentive and opportunity to live up to that trust and learn how to be trustworthy. When we think about it, this is a major part of what is involved in professional education and training, particularly during the periods of practical placements or work experience undertaken by trainee social workers and nurses. If trustworthiness in professional life involves being reliable, plausible and responsible at work, then supervised practice in doing particular tasks repeatedly (say inserting a naso-gastric tube or completing a community care assessment) encourages reliability in doing the tasks well; and doing the task alone at some later stage encourages the trainee also to take responsibility for the satisfactory completion of the task. If the tutor, supervisor or team manager has clear expectations of the trainee or professional practitioner, then this encourages the trainee to live up to these expectations.

Creating an organisational climate where trustworthiness is expected and valued

This follows on from the first point, but goes one stage further by situating the professional practitioner in an organisational context, which can be designed so as to have the effect of reinforcing the expectation of trustworthiness and facilitating its achievement. For example, in an organisation where there is no concept of team-working, where each individual practitioner looks out for themselves, many are fiddling their expenses and emotional abuse and neglect of patients or service users is occurring, the trustworthy person may struggle to maintain her high standards. Whereas in a strong team, where responsibility is shared and owned, there is a shared commitment to high standards, pride in the work and positive feedback from managers, colleagues and service users, it may be much easier to be trustworthy and to develop trustworthiness in practitioners. Similarly, in a climate of excessive regulation and surveillance, where practitioners' behaviour is controlled, there may be less incentive and fewer possibilities to be trustworthy.

Role modelling

This again is linked to the first two points and is a common strategy for developing all the virtues. Having available role models who behave in a trustworthy fashion is vital for helping develop trustworthy practitioners. This can be facilitated through encouraging students and practitioners to observe the behaviour and approach of others over time, as well as through experiencing themselves a trusting relationship with a trustworthy mentor.

Learning through role play and discussion of cases

The importance of being trustworthy and being regarded as trustworthy can also be experienced through role playing particular situations where trust is present or absent or can be discussed in relation to particular cases. For example, we might take the situation described by Lynne in the first vignette, with one person playing the paediatric nurse and the other the mother. The person taking on the role of Lynne could be asked to think very carefully about how to perform as a trustworthy nurse, and what it might feel like, initially, not to be trusted. The person taking on the role of the mother could try to imagine what it would be like to leave a seriously ill baby in the care of a new nurse, and how important it would be for the mother to regard the nurse as completely trustworthy. The role play could be varied and repeated on several occasions, with the person playing the nurse acting out the role of an untrustworthy nurse and the mother being played as a naïve or gullible person.

Concluding comments

Trustworthiness is not an easy quality to identify and abstract from other aspects of people's character or from the contexts in which people's behaviour and attitudes are located. In so far as it is embedded in the very definition of what it means to be a professional, then arguably trustworthiness shapes the nature of the professional role. A professional who is found to be untrustworthy in significant ways can no longer be regarded as a professional. Although we could say the same about any of the virtues, trustworthiness is perhaps more integral to the professional role than some of the others we examine in this book. A nurse or social worker who was relatively lacking in courage, respectfulness or care, for example, might just about get away with carrying out their professional role, albeit not very well; whereas a professional who was relatively lacking in trustworthiness could hardly be regarded as a professional at all. It is significant that in the judgements made in cases of professional misconduct, where professionals are removed from the register, reference to trust is frequently made. For example, in a case we use as a vignette in the chapter on integrity, about a nurse who falsified research data and was removed from the nursing register, the reasons given were 'breach of trust', and 'her actions undermined trust and confidence in the professions' (Nursing and Midwifery Council (NMC), 2004a, p. 13). This last point acknowledges the importance of professionals not only being trustworthy (behaving reliably and responsibly), but being regarded as trustworthy (being able to perform plausibly and publicly as reliable and responsible people).

Chapter 8

Justice

Introduction

'Justice' in contemporary moral philosophy is often associated with principle-based approaches to ethics, as opposed to those based on character or relationships. Indeed, 'justice' is one of the four core principles identified by Beauchamp and Childress (2001) in their influential text on biomedical ethics, and by many others who develop similar sets of principles for health and social care. There are, however, extensive accounts of justice as a virtue or moral quality, both of individuals and of social institutions. Aristotle and Plato give detailed analyses of justice as a virtue, while Rawls (1973, p. 3) famously characterises justice as 'the first virtue of social institutions' We are more concerned in this chapter with justice as a virtue of individuals, although we will argue that justice as an individual virtue and justice as a virtue of social institutions are inter-connected, in that just individuals are concerned to promote just social arrangements.

After discussing two vignettes, we will then consider different conceptions of justice (as a universal virtue and a particular virtue; a virtue of individuals and of social institutions; as distributive, retributive, reparative, restorative or transformative). We will suggest how justice in all these senses is about fair allocation of goods and harms, requiring practical wisdom in assessing particular cases in the light of laws, principles or rules and in developing, evaluating and critiquing laws, norms and existing social arrangements.

Vignettes

1) Being fair in distributing resources: a nurse's account

This extract is taken from an interview with the paediatric nurse, Lynne, whose example about trustworthiness we used in Chapter 7. When asked her views on justice, this is what she said:

> I think it's about *being fair*. I mean I can remember trying to send, or arranging to send, quite poorly children home, to parents who wanted them at home but they needed to have certain things set up at home before they could go – you know, piped oxygen and agency nurses coming in to help relieve them for the care of the child. And having to go to a commissioning meeting where the health authority was going to decide whether they were going to pay however much for the child. The person who came from the health authority, I know she has only a small pot of money really so she has to decide *how to sort of spread it out as best as possible*. But it seemed to me that this child should be allowed the opportunity to go home, so we really had to fight a case on the value of the child going home and had to know what sort of care the child was going to require. I mean there was a lot of people there, I mean the child's GP and different people from the ward, so I think it was a lot to do with negotiating, putting our facts across and being quite factual as well. I mean getting emotional, although we all felt emotional about child […] that wouldn't have got us anywhere. So we had to look at it *in a very black and white way* because that was the way the commissioner from the health authority looked at it. I mean this was *just another child who needed help* when it went home, if it went home. So we had to come at it almost from the same angle, I think, so that the child was able to go home and got *what we thought was fair* really. (Source: interview. Our italics)

2) Working with a Sikh family: perspectives from a social work supervisor

This vignette is taken from an interview with a senior social worker, James, who supervises a number of social work students during their fieldwork practice periods. The agency where James is based is located in a culturally diverse area of a large British city. James explained that about 70 per cent of the families they work with are from minority ethnic communities, mainly Sikh and Muslim. So the agency provides a challenging learning environment, particularly for white students who have to 'work cross-culturally' and need to consider 'cultural norms' and examine 'their own prejudice'. He described the work of a white male student who was working with a Sikh family, one member of which was a 21-year old young man with moderate learning difficulties and mental health problems. James described the young man as very withdrawn, prone to periods of long depression and quite 'monosyllabic'. The student had done excellent work both in getting the young man to be more communicative and in working with his father.

The agency had worked with the young man for the last five to six years. Before the student had got involved, the agency had only had contact with one parent, the mother. The student had spent a lot of time with the father and managed to engage him in thinking about the care of his son. James described a recent 'crisis' in this case, which had involved the young man in a fraças in the local park. James was aware of some of the details of this incident as he had been observing the student's practice during a meeting between a solicitor, the student and the young man's father. James's account is as follows:

This young man had never been in problems with the police before and he had gone into the local park and some young teenage girls had started calling him names both around his disability and also racist names [   ] I think these girls are about 14 or 15, and then I think he'd chased after them and they'd shouted more and then the allegation was that he had punched one of the girls and they went to the police and he was then charged with breaching the peace and assault. And I think it was the very nature of that had [caused] this sort of crisis. This is the first time, I mean when I was in this meeting the father was quite distressed and he said: 'I've lived in this house for 20 years, we've never been in any trouble'. And he said: 'When the police came, they didn't need to, and they put handcuffs on him and they took my son away in handcuffs and the neighbours were all looking and thinking: "Why is my son being taken off?" '. He didn't need to be, he's not aggressive, he wouldn't resist arrest, he didn't need to be treated, I mean he's a very vulnerable young man.

So I think [...] there was a kind of sense of being, their reputation being sullied and humiliated, you know, and so I think it was the nature of the crisis that had really precipitated that involvement. He'd also been locked up in the cells overnight and he alleges that he was kicked and water was thrown over him in the cells. So the student is then looking with the family at *taking out a complaint* against the police, you know, this is a vulnerable young man and particularly the police in this area are looking [at what they are doing] in terms of their race relations and this certainly doesn't help [...]

But I think also for the father to be believed, and then to see that this was a student, who [...] could take action and *advocate on their behalf.* I think on reflection now that was important and that he acknowledged his distress at what he felt was a humiliation of his son being arrested.

James discussed further details of the work the agency had done with this young man, including responding to the parents' concern that he should be placed in some kind of employment. But this was difficult to achieve, as James explained there was an issue about:

What resources are available. Because in so many ways *he was discriminated against on lots of levels*: he was black, he had a learning disability and he had mental health problems. And we would find that there would be services set up for people with mental health problems, but couldn't cope with somebody who was black or had a learning difficulty. And then the learning difficulty services might not be ethnically sensitive and couldn't cope with the mental health. So it's actually trying to find a resource that could offer some support and employment that could take account of these factors. Obviously then with the police charge [...] if he has a record then that is going to [have a] further impact so *he's going to be discriminated against on lots of levels or disadvantaged* potentially.
(Source: interview. Our italics)

Reflections

In the first vignette, after talking about children in general, Lynne shifts to a particular case. From what she says, we get the impression that she was quite emotionally engaged with the care of a particular child. However, in the context of being involved in decision-making about home care requirements, she then steps back from the case and views the child she is concerned about as just one among many children who need resources. She appreciates the position of the commissioner from the health authority, who has a small amount of money and needs to spread it out as fairly as possible. So we might characterise the situation as one where Lynne moves her focus from her caring relationship with this particular child and family to a more impartial perspective, seeing this child as 'just another child who needed help when it went home'. She even refers to the child as 'it' at this point, which depersonalises the relationship. It is not quite clear from the account Lynne gives to what extent she adopts an impartial approach because she knows this will gain the resources for the child (rather than emotionality or special pleading); or whether it is because she herself believes this is the way to be fair. Lynne ends the story by saying that the child was able to go home and 'got what we thought was fair really'. Although Lynne does not give explicit details, we could interpret this comment as entailing that the child was allocated enough resources to enable her to be cared for adequately at home (that is, to meet her needs), without taking up an excessive share of the limited resources (that is, not preventing others in need from benefiting in the future).

Lynne's account focuses more on the process of making a fair (or 'just') decision and obtaining a fair outcome, than on what it takes to be a 'just person'. However, since Lynne equates justice with 'being fair' and she attributes to the commissioner from the health authority the stimulus for the process of reaching what was ultimately a fair outcome, the commissioner could be regarded as personifying justice in the sense of working to ensure a fair distribution of goods between people. The commissioner is a neutral arbiter, with no special connection to any of the children herself, who needs to know factual information. She is in the position analogous to that of a judge in a legal case. Lynne, who starts off seemingly as an advocate of the child, seems almost herself to move into a neutral position in order to speak the language of justice.

The second vignette is based on an account from a social worker of work that he is supervising, in this case, that of a student, rather than work in which he is directly involved. This is an important perspective to consider, as someone who has a supervisory or managerial position often has an overview of many aspects of the work and the context in which it is located – for example, service users' needs in general, the quality of a range of practitioners' work, the role of the service-providing agency and the way policy impacts on practice. So issues of fairness, resource allocation and discrimination might be expected to feature in such an account, which is further removed from the minutiae of day-to-day practice. James does not actually use the terms 'justice' or 'fairness', but he does describe the discrimination faced by people from minority ethnic backgrounds, people with learning disabilities and mental health problems and the challenges faced by the young Sikh man who has all these characteristics. The way the account is given suggests that both James and the student he is supervising regard the treatment by the police of the young man as not only inappropriate, but as a case of negative discrimination. It is this interpretation of the situation that has prompted the student (with James's support) to act as an advocate on behalf of the family, helping them to make a complaint about the police actions.

In contrast to Lynne's position in the first vignette (when she moved towards taking the perspective of 'judge'), the social work student and supervisor, having heard about what they regard as unfair treatment, then decide to take up a position of offering support to the young man as a 'victim' of negative discrimination (acting as an advocate, in a position analogous to a lawyer acting for one party in a court case). Here the issue of the powerlessness and vulnerability of the service user is a key underlying theme. The Sikh family is presented as victim, therefore needing support to challenge the insensitive and discriminatory attitudes and actions of the police, which are part of endemic and widespread discrimination (direct and indirect) in services and in society generally. This is not to imply that the young women in the park, one of whom was alleged to have been assaulted, are not also 'victims' in this case. However, since the police were pursuing their case, the social workers focussed their attention on the young Sikh man as their 'client', with whom they already have a supporting role.

Conceptions of justice

Whilst all the concepts and virtues we discuss in the book are both complex and contested, justice seems particularly so in that it has several different meanings informed by different theoretical and ideological positions. Although we are concerned in this chapter primarily with justice as a moral quality of individuals (that is, justice as an individual virtue), this cannot be divorced from social justice (that is, justice as a virtue of social institutions). Indeed the second vignette shows how the social worker, James, sees what he regards as the unjust behaviour of the police as located in unjust social institutions. Debates about the latter, in particular what counts as just social arrangements, have exercised philosophers, politicians and other thinkers and policy-makers from ancient times to the present day. Hence the terrain that has been travelled in pursuing the question 'What is justice?' is wide, deep and criss-crossed with many twisting, diverging and overlapping paths.

In addition to the distinction between justice as a virtue of individuals and justice as a virtue of social institutions, there are also broader and narrower conceptions of justice as a virtue of individuals. Using Aristotle's terms, we may distinguish between particular justice (as one virtue among several) and universal justice (as a kind of overarching virtue encompassing the whole of morality). It is the former that interests us here (that is, justice as one moral quality alongside others such as care, respectfulness and so on). However, the fact that some people have articulated a broader sense of justice is significant, as this inevitably colours our view of justice as a particular virtue. It is here that we will start our discussion of justice.

Universal justice

Arguably both the vignettes we have chosen to illustrate justice include measuring the needs and/or rights of one individual in comparison with others. So there is an element of detachment or impartiality involved. Although both also feature partiality (a coming close to the individual concerned in order to assess their needs, and an element of emotional commitment to getting the best for the individuals concerned), for these vignettes to be about justice (rather than care or respectfulness, for example), it is the features of measurement, comparison and overview that are important. Given many philosophers and other theorists see impartiality and detachment as a key feature of morality, then we should not be surprised if justice is seen either as an overarching virtue or as a key organising principle for making moral judgements. We will focus here on virtue ethical accounts of justice. But it is worth noting that principle-based accounts of ethics also feature this broad sense of justice (encapsulated in, for example, Kohlberg's (1981, 1984) influential account of morality, which has often been termed an ethic(s) of justice, in that the higher stages of morality are equated with this kind of impartiality and detachment).

Both Aristotle and Plato offer substantial virtue ethical accounts of justice that are so all-encompassing as to include the whole of morality. Aristotle (1954, 1128b35–1129a23) suggests there are two senses of justice: universal ('the lawful') and particular ('the fair'). It is universal justice, which he equates with 'the lawful', that Aristotle claims amounts to 'complete virtue'. While today we would not equate just acts with lawful acts in the way Aristotle does (that is, we do think the law can be unjust), we need to appreciate Aristotle's view of the law as comprehensive, commanding that citizens act in accordance with all the virtues (bravery, temperateness, good temper and so on) and forbidding forms of wickedness. Justice, he claims, is about exercising virtue in relations with our neighbours. This explains why he claims (p. 108) that justice in this sense is often thought to be the greatest of the virtues:

> 'Neither evening nor morning star' is so wonderful; and proverbially 'in justice is every virtue comprehended'. And it is complete virtue in its fullest sense because it is the actual exercise of complete virtue.

Plato's conception of justice, as expounded in the *Republic*, is somewhat different, but similarly all-embracing, in that he defines justice as harmony in the soul. He depicts justice in the state as a situation when each of the other three cardinal virtues (wisdom, courage and discipline/temperance) is doing the job for which it is naturally fitted and not interfering with the others. Justice in the individual mirrors justice in the state, so that an individual is just, according to Plato, in respect of the harmony that exists when all three elements of the mind perform their proper function and so achieve their proper fulfilment (Plato, 1955, pp 193–194).

Particular justice

Both these conceptions of justice see it as a kind of overarching virtue, although for Aristotle it is about promoting just social arrangements, whilst for Plato it is an internal state of mind (Slote, 2002, p. 2). Aristotle's second sense of justice, however, is particular justice or 'justice as value'. This is a singular virtue, which is a part of 'complete virtue' alongside the other virtues such as respectfulness, courage and so on. According to Aristotle this comprises 'the just as the fair and equal' or 'justice as equity'. Within this conception of justice as one of the virtues, Aristotle (1954: 1130a6–1131a6) distinguishes between distributive and rectificatory justice. Distributive justice is concerned with the distribution of honour or money or 'other things that fall to be divided among those who have a share in the constitution' in accordance with geometrical proportions, while rectificatory justice plays a rectifying part in human transactions, such as sales, loans, thefts, assaults or insults (in accordance with arithmetical progression). Aristotle's account of different kinds of justice suggests that it is not a unitary concept, even when conceived as a singular virtue.

It is also very common in contemporary writings to distinguish distributive justice (often used in the context of discussions of social justice, that is, just social arrangements for promoting welfare, health and so on) from justice in the context of individual exchange and meting out of compensation or punishment (rectificatory, restorative or retributive). Nevertheless, 'distribution', broadly conceived, does seem to be involved in both types of justice. Clearly 'distribution' (in the general sense of a process of allocation or re-allocation of goods and harms between people) is at the core of all versions of justice, alongside some form of calculation in order to decide on what is a 'fair' distribution/allocation. However, to avoid confusion, it is important to note this more specialist use of the term 'distribution' to refer to the allocation of benefits and burdens amongst a range of people, often as part of social policy. Therefore we will tend to use the term 'allocation' as a more neutral, all-encompassing term, applying to both 'distributive' and 'rectificatory' justice.

The contestability of justice

The fact that there are both universal and particular conceptions of justice and different types of particular justice is not the only source of confusion. MacIntyre (1985, pp. 244–255), in *After Virtue*, devotes a chapter to justice, demonstrating the lack of consensus in contemporary society about the nature of justice as a particular virtue. Although he does not explicitly state this, he is, in fact, concerned with distributive justice, as described above. He outlines the cases put by two fictional characters for justice based on entitlement (to property and income legitimately gained and earned) and for justice based on equality in meeting needs (hence leading to redistribution of property and income to the most needy). These two claims approximate to the conceptions of justice put forward by Nozick (1974), who espouses a libertarian view of justice (based on individual entitlements and freedom), and Rawls (1973), who espouses a kind of liberal egalitarianism (based on minimal levels of equality for all). MacIntyre argues that these two types of claims are incommensurable, that is, they are not measurable in terms of a common standard and hence cannot be weighed against each other. He sees this as exemplifying an inability to agree upon the content and character of particular virtues.

While we might agree with MacIntyre that Nozick and Rawls have different conceptions of what counts as just social arrangements, what they have in common is a concern with fair allocation of property and other distributable goods. What they disagree about, of course, is what counts substantively as a 'fair' allocation of goods and how this can be achieved. Whilst MacIntyre only offers two accounts of justice, he acknowledges that there are many more (including justice as desert, for example). This is illustrated by Beauchamp and Childress (1994, pp. 329–331) in their book on biomedical ethics, where they identify six 'material principles' of distributive justice. Whilst their account is principle-based, these principles clearly relate to the conception of and the commitment to justice that would inform a virtue ethics account of justice. These are that distribution should occur to each person according to: equal shares; need; effort; contribution; merit; or free market exchanges. They suggest that some theories of justice accept all six principles as valid. They also argue that each principle identifies a prima facie obligation, the weight of which should be assessed in the context of the particular circumstances or spheres in which they are especially applicable. We could interpret this as meaning that, for example, when allocating marks to students in the context of formal academic examinations, merit is usually used as a criterion; while in allocating health and social care services, need is often predominant. There may, of course, be some debate over what should be used as a fair principle (some might argue that account should be taken of effort in children's examinations; or that merit and free-market principles should come into health care). We would question, however, whether this disagreement is necessarily as problematic as MacIntyre suggests.

For some philosophers, such a clash of interpretations may be welcomed as part of our complex human fate. Ricoeur (2007, p. 62), for example, in his account of justice, sees it ultimately as to do with making fair decisions: 'the difficult decisions that have to be made in circumstances marked by incertitude and conflict under the sign of the tragic dimension of action'. What counts as 'fair' has to be assessed in the context of each situation. A 'just' person could be described as one who thinks about, and assesses carefully, which criteria (desert, need and so on) are most appropriate and how they should be applied in the allocation of goods and harms in the overall scheme of promoting human flourishing. This suggests that being just is inextricably linked with practical wisdom. While each case or situation is different, cases similar in relevant respects also need to be treated similarly – so it is important to have a set of criteria, principles or rules for allocation. These will need to be interpreted in each situation, as a judge in a law court interprets the law in relation to each case. This does not mean that the rules, principles or laws are not open to critical challenge. Indeed, a sense of justice may cause us to challenge the law (for example, the death penalty in some states of the USA or laws on immigration and asylum in many northern countries). As Comte-Sponville (2003, p. 63) points out, laws are made by the majority, not the most just. We can distinguish the law as fact (legality) from the law as value (legitimacy).

MacIntyre's point that we do not share a common conception of justice because we do not share a common conception of the good (or what counts as human flourishing) applies equally, of course, to all the virtues and leads him to develop his account of virtues as relative to particular communities and practices. So his critique is not specific to justice. However, justice is a particularly good example of a virtue about which there is substantial disagreement as to its moral content. For even though we have included it as one of our substantive moral virtues (that is, it does have moral content; it is not simply a way of organising the other virtues), it is very hard to pin down the substantive content.

Justice and impartiality

If we reflect more deeply on justice, particularly as depicted in the first (nursing) vignette, it does seem a rather different type of moral concept and virtue to the other substantive virtues. Care, respectfulness and trustworthiness all have a focus on the nature and quality of the relationships between people. They entail a kind of communicative engagement or recognition on the part of the caring, respectful or trustworthy person. Justice, as depicted here, seems to have some features of what we have described as 'structural' virtues in that it has quite a strong focus on the distribution or allocation of goods and harms and the making of calculative comparisons between people – hence the importance of impartiality.

Having said this, on first reading, the second (social work) vignette may seem to depict a somewhat different conception of justice – as the attitudes and behaviour of the social workers, based on non-discriminatory and positively discriminatory treatment of the Sikh family, do seem to be based on a relationship between them and the family. Indeed, some commentators might argue that this vignette is not really about 'justice', if impartiality is thought to be the core of justice. However, another way of viewing the second vignette is to say that that the attitudes and behaviours of the social workers described encompass justice, alongside and intertwined with care and respectfulness. Most of the relationship work that would go into treating the young Sikh man 'positively' would require the qualities of care and respectfulness. In particular, it would entail that version of respect that encompasses recognition for difference in culture, religion, physical and mental capacities (Williams, 2000). 'Justice' comes in when the professionals start to make a kind of calculation or assessment of, for example, whether the young man deserves to be treated in the way he apparently was by the police, with reference to his capacities and his needs, compared with other people. Nevertheless, the conception of justice in the second vignette, which is based on social workers recognising and valuing differences between this young man and other people and identifying his specific needs, is rather different from the process the nurse goes through in the first vignette, of standing back and seeing the baby in question as just one baby among many in similar circumstances. If we want to connect this with the broader literature on recognition (of cultural differences) and redistribution (of social and economic goods), then we could say that in the case of the

Sikh young man we are talking about 'recognition' and in the case of deciding which babies should go home from hospital, we are talking about (re)distribution. Although there is ongoing debate about the relationship between these two concepts and the political philosophies on which they are based (Fraser and Honneth, 2003; Honneth, 2001), it seems clear to us that they are inextricably intertwined.

However, what we have been discussing above are the *processes* by which to achieve justice – by standing back, or coming close – and these may vary according to the situation. Lynne already had close contact with the baby in her care, so she stood back in order to see this baby's needs in perspective. The police in the second vignette would initially be distant from the young man, which is why the social workers felt they should put the young man's particular needs and circumstances into the frame. Do these vignettes necessarily embody different conceptions of justice? Or is one about recognition of difference rather than justice as (re)distribution? Both are about meeting individuals' needs in the context of the relevant needs/interests of a wide range of others. This requires knowing the individual, as well as having the wider picture. The conception(s) of justice embodied in both these vignettes seem to be about 'fair allocation of benefits and burdens'. In both vignettes the professionals telling the story could be interpreted as regarding 'fair' as taking account of individual needs – with the issue being how to place this in a broader institutional or societal context where the needs of a large number of others are at stake too. This raises the question of the relationship between individual and social justice mentioned earlier. Slote (2002) distinguishes justice as an individual virtue (that is, a quality of individual people) from social justice (a virtue of institutions). Clearly it is the former that interests us here, whereas it is the latter that is the focus of attention of the accounts of justice given by political philosophers such as Rawls (1973, 1993), Nozick (1974), Sandel (1998) and Walzer (1983), whose focus is on the nature of just social arrangements.

However, justice as a virtue of an individual person is, it seems to us, not unrelated to social justice. If we define the virtue of justice very inclusively as a disposition to act justly in all circumstances, then justice will include, as Adams (2006, p. 183) suggests:

Treating others as one owes it to them to do, respecting their rights, and upholding or promoting just causes or institutions.

That is, justice comprises a disposition to act fairly in relation to individuals to whom one owes a particular obligation and to act in a way that promotes and reflects just social arrangements. While some commentators suggest justice (as impartial distribution) is not a virtue in the traditional Aristotelian sense as 'its place in the overall blueprint for individual flourishing remains obscure' (Cottingham, 1996, pp. 68–69), arguably, the sense of 'flourishing' that forms part of professional ethics (linked with public good) can easily accommodate justice as a virtue.

Justice as restorative and transformative

The association of the concept of justice with 'impartiality' (as depicted in the first vignette) is very common. This is epitomised, as Phillips (2004, p. 110) points out, in the Roman goddess of justice (*Justitia*), who is often depicted on flags or in statues in front of courthouses as blindfolded and holding two balanced scales:

> Her blindfold and the scales she holds symbolise her ability to judge both the powerful and the powerless without bias, and to carry out the law without prejudice.

Phillips gives an account of a contemporary Socratic dialogue he facilitated in Mexico on the theme of 'What is justice?' He records how, after one participant suggested that justice should be 'blind' and non-preferential, like the statue of Justitia, another participant, a woman, said:

> I don't want justice to be blind at all ... I want justice to be applied with her eyes open to the oppression and wrongs we've suffered.

This woman then recounted how her cousin was arrested in 1968 for participating in pro-democracy protests and along with many others was tortured until he died. Those who committed these crimes were never named or punished. The current president of Mexico has finally agreed that there should be a 'truth commission' to find out what happened. It is interesting that the term 'truth' is used in this context, rather than 'justice'. This is because the main concern is to find out and document what actually happened. As with the more well-known example in South Africa (The Truth and Reconciliation Commission), in so far as such commissions are concerned with justice it is reparative or restorative justice – that is, the recognising of past wrongs, repairing or restoring of relationships, forgiveness, learning from past mistakes and moving on. As Ricoeur (2007, pp. 69–70) points out in his essay on 'Justice and Truth', in the legal sphere two parallel processes are happening: the interpretation of the facts of what happened (a narrative process) and juridical reasoning about the law (application of the norm to the case). In restorative or reparative justice we may be as concerned with the former as the latter. This is distinct from both redistributive justice (for example, offering compensation) and retributive justice (for example, punishment commensurate with the harm caused). Nevertheless in all forms of justice the person in the position of 'judge' needs the capacity to negotiate between the personal (partial) and the impersonal (impartial) points of view. As full a story (or set of stories) as possible is required in order that an impartial judgement can be made. If we are to see justice as a mean, then it lies between excessive partiality or emotional involvement, and extreme indifference or arrogance. As Ricoeur (2007, p. 61) says, 'the quest for justice is for a just distance among all human beings'.

If we take restorative justice further, placing more of a focus on the future than the past, it may develop into what some have termed 'transformative' justice (Phillips, 2004, p. 140), which includes a commitment to eliminate endemic inequalities. While the social worker in the second vignette is not explicitly advocating transformative justice, his analysis of the shortcomings in the social care and police services suggests a belief in a better society where such inequalities are eradicated. This kind of commitment is evident in some of the community and social work literature, in which professional work is explicitly framed as working for transformative change towards social justice (for example: Adams, Dominelli and Payne, 2005; Butcher, Banks, Henderson and Robertson, 2007; Dominelli, 2002; Hope and Timmel, 1999). It is important, therefore, to take account of transformative justice in any discussion of the individual virtue of justice. Often when we talk of a 'just person', we are referring to someone who has a disposition to act fairly in particular situations (to calculate carefully how to allocate goods and harms, based on sound criteria) and to promote and maintain fair social arrangements within the broad boundaries of the current social system. This would apply to the health commissioner in the first vignette. However, what if the

health commissioner regards the current system of resource allocation as unfair? Let us assume that the budget for paediatric nursing
has been cut recently in order to redeploy nursing staff as part of a
strategy to reduce the waiting times for minor operations. We might
expect a health commissioner with a sense of justice to challenge this
with those in charge of resource allocation, or indeed, with politicians responsible for health care policy. It is important that the moral
quality of justice includes transformative justice as a 'module'. As
with the other virtues, justice can be regarded as 'modular'. It is possible, therefore, for someone to be called 'just' if they are disposed to
act justly in certain sorts of circumstances: for example, if they pay
particular attention to fair allocation of goods within the status quo.
This person may not be inspired by a vision of a transformed society,
where greater material and social equality prevails. However, there
are other contexts where transformative justice is at stake – and in
health and social care it is important that we see the bigger picture
and are prepared to challenge the status quo, for which the virtue of
courage is required.

Strategies for practice and professional education

Developing the ability to assess needs and resources

In so far as justice is about ensuring a fair allocation of harms and
goods between people (and this may include potential people, as yet
unborn), then clearly just people require a great deal of practical wisdom. In particular, the just health or social care professional needs
to be able to see where issues of fairness arise in their work and
be able to weigh up and calculate what proportion of resources or
other goods should be allocated to particular individuals or groups.
Beginning practitioners often do not have an overview of the range
of work to be done, resources available and potential service user
demands. So it is easy to become closely involved with one patient
or service user, to give too much time or resources to someone who
shouts loudly or to focus on the needs of one individual in isolation from their family or wider community. Encouraging students
and beginning practitioners to stand back from their day-to-day
tasks, to analyse the role and resources of the agency/project/sec-
tion where they are working or to undertake an audit of current
and future needs are all ways of developing their abilities to see a

broader picture and to assess needs and resources (see Dickenson, 1994; Hardcastle, Powers and Wencour, 2004, Chapter 6, for a useful overview of approaches to community analysis).

Supervision can also be helpful in encouraging a practitioner to contextualise their work. While we might accept that it was a legitimate social work role for the student to advocate for the Sikh young man in the second vignette, in discussing the broader implications of the case in supervision, the supervisor might encourage the student to consider the position and perspective of the young women in the park. While the young women may need educating in order to develop a more respectful attitude to people who are different from themselves, it could be argued that they have the right to play in the park without being subject to assault. This adds further weight to arguments for improving services and support for people with learning disabilities and mental health problems, as well as anti-racist work with young people.

Developing political awareness and a critical approach to practice

Seeing the bigger picture also contributes to developing an awareness of the contribution of politics and policy to the context in which health and social care practice takes place. There is a sense in which just practitioners need to be critical practitioners – with the theoretical and practical resources to reflect on practice, to locate the sources and influence of power, to see their own roles as contributing to the perpetuation of injustice and oppression and with the commitment and competence to work creatively for social change. Research by one of the authors on community-based practitioners identifies several features that are relevant here. According to Banks (2007), the critical practitioner is prepared to move beyond the 'comfort zone'; has a clear and strong belief in a set of professional values (which may entail being 'passionate' about social justice, or 'righteously angry' about injustice); critical self-awareness and reflexivity; and the capacity to put values into practice (practical wisdom and praxis).

Role modelling

A senior practitioner or teacher has the potential to serve as a role model for inexperienced, trainee or student practitioners. This would involve being careful not to show unwarranted favouritism or neglect towards particular students or service users and ensuring those who are vulnerable, less vocal or who have greater needs gain attention or resources. Observations of senior practitioners making assessments, of case conferences and team meetings where cases are allocated or resource decisions made, all provide useful experience. Key figures who have campaigned tirelessly for social justice in the past or present, both inside and outside the profession, can also serve as a source of inspiration – from Augustus Barnett and Jane Addams (pioneers of work in socially disadvantaged areas) to Florence Nightingale and Nelson Mandela.

Practising decision-making and advocacy

Inexperienced or trainee practitioners can be encouraged to make decisions themselves about allocating resources, with the possibility of talking through their options in supervision. Having to take on an advocacy role, like the social work student in the second vignette, encourages the thinking through of how to make a case for special needs and resources. The use of practice placement periods to undertake real and responsible work, well supported, is crucial to helping trainee and beginning practitioners to develop a sense of justice and to rehearse how to make decisions and take action.

Learning through role play and discussion of cases

As with the other virtues, a feeling for the nature and importance of justice can be developed through discussing particular cases in class or learning sets, or through role play. In health and social care the limited resources available compared with the potential or actual demand and need is very great. While the decision about allocation of resources is frequently made by a manager or a panel or team, the frontline practitioner often has to make a recommendation or argue a case (as did Lynne in the first vignette). A scenario could be developed from the first vignette involving several babies currently in a hospital who could all go home, provided agency nurses were put in place. However, the budget for agency nursing is limited and is insufficient to allow all the babies to be discharged. Each one has different needs and home circumstances. How will it be decided which babies get the agency nursing? Discussing what criteria to use to make a fair decision, or role playing a multi-disciplinary team meeting, will encourage a debate about what counts as 'fair' and the testing out in group discussion of the implications of applying different criteria. The second vignette could also be developed to add in the perspectives of the two young women who first taunted and verbally abused the young Sikh man, and then were assaulted by him. Discussion could focus on how justice could be achieved for all parties, and whether it should be retributive, restorative or transformative. A second meeting between the young man and two young women, with a restorative aim in mind, would be an interesting scenario to act out.

Concluding comments

The very existence of state-supported systems of health and social care is based on some kind of commitment to just social arrangements (amongst other reasons such as maintaining social order and ensuring a healthy workforce). The design of such social arrangements is worked on and achieved by just individuals, as is the day-to-day implementation of just policies and practices. Whilst there is considerable debate about the substantive nature of individual and social justice, we have suggested that a common feature of all accounts is a concern with fair allocation of goods and harms between people (including future people) and, on some accounts, between all parts of the natural world. The virtue of justice requires practical wisdom, and often courage in taking action. Whilst we frequently focus attention on just individuals scrupulously following rules in the fair allocation of goods, within health and social care a commitment to transformative justice is equally important. This requires a critical stance to the work and an ability and commitment to challenge unjust social arrangements and work towards a society, and indeed a world, where goods and harms are more equally distributed.

Chapter 9

Courage

Introduction[1]

Courage is one of the most admired of the virtues. It is a very necessary virtue in professional practice, associated with responses to everyday and extreme fears. We typically associate courage with endurance and fortitude, with confronting fear and acting ethically in the face of individual and institutional vulnerability and fallibility. Courage is, primarily, a virtue associated with resilience and resistance

In health and social care practice professionals have to respond to a wide-range of fear-inducing situations. Interactions with service users may evoke fears of failure, of violence, of extreme emotional reactions, fears of contamination, of disclosing uncertainty, of making mistakes and of litigation. Encounters with colleagues and managers may evoke fears of disapproval, of losing face or of losing one's position. Adhering to the guidelines of professional codes often requires courage but this is not made explicit.

This chapter considers courage from a virtue perspective in the context of everyday practice. We argue that there are different types of courage – some moral and some non-moral – and that whereas modules of courage may be demonstrated, it is composite courage to which professionals need to aspire.

---

[1] Some of the material in this chapter draws on an unpublished PhD thesis (Gallaghar 2003).

Vignettes

1) Having the courage to knock on the door: a social worker's story

Jeremy is an experienced social worker specialising in safeguarding children in a local authority children's service. When asked about the role of courage in relation to his social work practice, he talked about the challenges of home visits. He said the question 'How hard should I knock?' was sometimes not far from mind. Here Jeremy describes his experience of visiting families that he was assigned to investigate, recalling one particular family:

> I'd read the file, and it mentioned a history of violence, and I had to go round to talk to them about some bruising which day nursery staff had found on their child.
>
> First off, how should I try not to look like a social worker? My car was not a good start as it was obviously more expensive than anything else in the street. My clothes also suggested that I was 'official'. I wasn't sure if I should carry a briefcase or notepad or nothing. I'd need to take notes and I was worried about leaving my diary in the car as it contained information about other clients.
>
> I struggled more generally with my identity as a social worker on such visits. On the one hand, I was committed to the view that I was promoting the well-being of service users I work with. But, on the other hand, I was acutely aware of the importance of child protection and the power I had in the process of removing children from their parents to put them into care or submit reports that could incriminate someone resulting in imprisonment.
>
> So when I went on a home visit I was aware that I might not be welcome and might even be assaulted. This was a time when the statistics were showing that pro rata more social workers were killed whilst working than police officers. I was also aware of findings from investigations into child protection failures and realised the importance of making contact with families. Nevertheless, sometimes I did consider how hard do I have to knock to be able to write, truthfully, on the file: 'Visited – no reply'? We used to joke about it – 'knocking on the door with a damp sponge'.
> (Source: interview)

2) Having the courage to say 'this is not right': speaking up about unacceptable practice

The second example is unlike others in this book. It comes from an Irish government report, *The Lourdes Hospital Inquiry: An Inquiry into Peripartum Hysterectomy at Our Lady of Lourdes Hospital, Drogheda* (Harding Clark, 2006).[2] In this report the Irish High Court Judge, Maureen Harding Clark, details events leading up to, and following, a verdict of professional misconduct and the striking off the medical register of the obstetrician and gynaecologist, Dr Michael Neary, in 2003. It was established that an unacceptably high rate of peripartum hysterectomies (an operation to remove the womb within six weeks of giving birth) had been performed at the Lourdes hospital over the 25-year period that Dr Neary was employed as a consultant there. Dr Neary's practice was not subject to scrutiny until October 1998 when two experienced midwives sought the advice of the Health Board solicitor regarding their concerns.

The Harding Clark Report (2006) provides different perspectives on the role and implications of fear and courage. The inquiry team stated that they 'had difficulty understanding why so few had the courage, insight, curiosity or integrity to say "this is not right"' (p. 316). The report introduction and overview states that:

> We uncovered a complex story, and many strands remain tangled in the personalities of the participants and the difficult relationship between religious beliefs and human reproduction overlaid with a sense of intense loyalty to the Maternity Unit. It is a story set in a time of unquestioning submission to authority, whether religious or civil, when nurses and doctors were in abundant supply and permanent jobs were few and treasured. The MMMs [the Medical Missionaries of Mary – an order of Catholic nuns] ran a very ordered hospital in an austere and dedicated manner. (p. 29)

---

[2] We are grateful to Joan McCarthy for bringing this report to our attention. Reproduced under Licence from The Stationery Office, Dublin. Extracts are reproduced from Harding Clark (2006) *The Lourdes Hospital Inquiry – An inquiry into Peripartum Hysterectomy at Our Lady of Lourdes Hospital Drogheda*, Dublin: The Stationery Office.

And

> The story of Dr. Neary's fall from grace is one of enormous trag-
> edy for the hospital at which he worked for 25 years, for the staff
> who work with and supported him and especially for the women
> who entered the maternity hospital to face the joy of a new baby
> and who returned home to recuperate from a hysterectomy. It has
> also had a profound affect on Dr. Neary's life, and on his family.
> This is not a simple story of an evil man or a bad doctor, nor is it
> the story of wholesale suppression of facts. There was no attempt
> to hide the procedures or pretend they were something else. The
> operations were carried out in the presence of consultant anaes-
> thetists, assisted at by trainee obstetricians who had all the text-
> books available to them and frequently observed by spouses and
> partners. The operations were openly recorded. (p. 34)

Different views and interpretations of the character and conduct of Dr
Neary are presented in the report. Some describe him as kind, caring
and hard-working while others describe him as crude, rude, abrupt
and opinionated. It is suggested that Dr Neary was frightened of
haemorrhage and engaged in defensive practice. The report discusses
the need to 'update Dr Neary in modern obstetric practice' and

> remedy the defects in his judgement, especially in relation to his
> abnormal reaction to haemorrhage [. . .] one member of the review
> body was quite confident that retraining would have produced
> appropriate results although he admitted that Dr Neary would
> have to change his belief that each hysterectomy was lifesaving
> and develop some insight into his propensity to exaggerate dan-
> ger. (p. 291)

The Medical Missionaries of Mary and the Catholic Church influenced surgical practices and nurse training. The report states:

> The sisters belonged to an era when nurses were efficient,
> ordered and respectful. They carried out orders and did not ques-
> tion consultants. Matron maintained a formal, distant authority
> over nurses. The nuns who had set the practices and protocols
> for training nurses and midwives in the 50s thus produced suit-
> able nurses and midwives who fitted the mould – hardworking,

respectful. Catholic nurses who were well trained, knew their place, trusted the consultants and suspended their critical or questioning faculties. They were trained to certain tasks – and to those tasks only. (p. 41)

It is, as Harding Clark points out, interesting to note that the midwives who spoke out had received their professional education elsewhere. (Source: Harding Clark, 2006)

3) Not falling apart – a paramedic's perspective

The third example is from a paramedic, Susan, who describes the role of courage in her everyday practice:

A lot of people come round and say 'I couldn't do your job, it must be really difficult' and I don't know if it's something you just have or you learn to deal with things as you go along. I suppose it's a way of dealing with things. No matter what kind of character you are you must have some kind of ability, to have courage under pressure or ... to be sort of a strong character when you need to be ... Just thinking of courage, ... I've done three paediatric resuses [resuscitations] in six or seven years. The youngest one was eighteen days old, and, if you're presented, at the front door with a mother who is holding their baby at arms length going 'help me' and this baby is obviously dead [...] You know in your heart that there is nothing you can do that will help this child even though you are going to go through everything that you possibly can. I think sometimes having the courage to do it even though you know it's, not worthless, but being able to deal with the situation and not falling apart for the mother's sake is sometimes really hard work. I think that kind of courage is not necessarily seeing severed limbs or lots of blood. I think that's where the courage comes in. It is more dealing with emotional problems, emotional difficulties, because you haven't got just the baby that you're trying to deal with in that situation, you've got a mother who is absolutely distraught [...]. All their faith and hope is in the ambulance that turns up and the hospital doctors and nurses that deal with the patients there. And you are the first person this mother sees and you've got to have courage so as not to fall apart completely in front of this mother because often I get asked 'what's the worst thing you've ever seen?', 'what's the most distressing?' And it's not the amputated legs, it's not the gunshot wounds or stab wounds, it's the completely distraught parent whose child is so unwell and you just, you know that, sometimes you know that you are trying to do your best but you're not sure that it's working. Other times, you know that it doesn't matter what you do, this child is not going to survive and you've got to put across the professionalness of knowing, of trying to show that you're doing everything you can, even though in your head you know it's worthless. That's, I think, where the courage comes in, not to fall apart from the emotional point of view, not from the horrendous physical injuries but more emotionally I think.

Susan describes one of the resuscitation attempts in more detail and gives reasons why the ambulance crew do not always adhere to protocol:

The first child, the eighteen-day-old one, was a cot death, had been dead for hours, there wasn't anything we could do. We'd been through full resuscitation. The reason you go through resuscitation, I mean obviously there's no reason to, we've got protocols to not start resus especially if they're obviously dead. So there are reasons not to start resus, but with this child the mother needs to get some kind of closure and often the best way is for them to understand that everything that could have been done was done so even though you look at this child and you think, you know, I've got no hope here, you're going to do as much as you can firstly, to convince yourself that you've done everything that you can, but also to try to reassure the mother that it was a terrible, you know, unfortunate incident. It wasn't anybody's fault; that everything was done that could have been done, so that she, the mother, can go away from that and think 'I did everything I could, I found my baby and I called an ambulance and they helped me and then the nursing staff, the hospital staff have helped me'. And even though the baby died, everybody helped. So that's probably, for those kind of jobs, it's more about convincing the mother you did everything you could, or the family, rather than actually doing any good for the child. It's more from an emotional, or from a mental point of view, for the mother, so maybe that's where the courage comes in [. . .]

A lot of other people, you know, need courage for approaching physical injuries but from my point of view, it's ill children. It's not that I can't cope with them, it's just that I have to muster up all my courage to deal, to be as professional as possible at the time and then not worry about falling apart afterwards.

(Source: interview)

Reflections

These three quite different examples provide insights and raise questions about the nature and role of courage within professional practice. The 'knocking with a damp sponge' vignette illustrates graphically the challenging nature of social work practice. Social workers have to respond to reports of harm and neglect within families and, when they do a home visit, often do not know what will transpire. Jeremy's account, he claims, refers to a time when more social workers were killed on duty than police officers, therefore, a fear of violence was reasonable.

Reticence about knocking is, to some extent, understandable and highlights a potential conflict between self-interest and the interests of others. Not knocking loudly enough may be self-protective for Jeremy as family members, if at home, will not be disturbed and the social worker will not experience anger or violence. Moreover, he can then leave a note saying he has called and record 'visited – no reply' which would, nominally, satisfy his professional obligations. However, given his awareness of child protection responsibilities (more commonly now referred to as 'safeguarding children') he appreciates the potentially serious implications of not trying harder to get a response. Fear of violence is a relevant consideration in Jeremy's account. He is aware of his own vulnerability and also of the vulnerability of the potentially endangered child(ren) and, perhaps also, adults if there is domestic violence or elder abuse.

Extracts from the Harding Clark Report (2006) provide insights into a health care situation where a high rate of peripartum hysterectomy went unchallenged for some 25 years. The report points out that the Lourdes Hospital story is not a simple one nor is it the story 'of an evil man or a bad doctor, nor is it the story of wholesale suppression of facts'. The extracts from the report suggest the significance of courage and fear. The midwives appeared to show courage in sharing their concerns at the risk of being labelled whistle-blowers, not having their contracts renewed or losing their jobs. Dr Neary was, the report suggests, afraid of haemorrhage and carried out unnecessary hysterectomies, while the Matron was afraid of being sued. These different examples suggest different fears and indicate the need for different types of courage.

The report also suggests, in common with other reports of inappropriate and unethical practices, the significance of institutional and professional cultures that make saying 'this is not right' difficult for professionals. The Public Inquiry into the care of children receiving complex cardiac surgery at Bristol Royal Infirmary (Kennedy, 2001), for example, pointed to failures in communication, in teamwork and leadership and to a 'club culture' where a few people had too much power and control. In such situations professionals may experience moral distress or feel unprepared to intervene.

In the third vignette, Susan talks of courage under pressure. For her, contrary to what many people might think, it is not the terrible injuries that people sustain that have the highest emotional impact, but rather not 'falling apart' in the presence of a 'distraught parent' when a child is gravely ill or dead. She describes how, in some situations, there is a need to demonstrate that the paramedic is 'doing everything you can' even if she is aware that this is futile. She talks of not acting in accordance with protocol to ensure that the parent has 'closure'.

The three examples suggest different types of courage, different degrees of courage, different behavioural dispositions and reasons why professionals might find it difficult to be courageous. They suggest how fear and courage present differently in everyday professional practice. Jeremy, for example, appears to fear violence and also the consequences of non-intervention. The midwives and other professionals in Drogheda may have feared being criticised and isolated, losing their jobs or being sued. Some spoke out despite these fears. Dr Neary, it seems, feared losing a patient due to haemorrhage. Susan focuses on the emotional aspect of courage in dealing with parents, suggesting perhaps the fear of not being able to hold it together and of not being able to show that everything possible is being done even if this is futile. The examples also suggest the role of other virtues in addition to courage. The Harding Clark report, for example, refers to curiosity and integrity. Susan refers to the role of hope and her discussion suggests also the role of professional wisdom.

Courage as a virtue

Courage is required in our everyday and professional lives. People are vulnerable to many actual and imaginary dangers and fear accompanies almost every developmental phase: fear as we learn to walk, fear as sexuality is awakened, fear as family responsibilities are assumed, fear as we grow old and anticipate death (Casey, 1990). These examples suggest a diverse range of fears that may be experienced in professional practice. A dictionary definition states that courage originates from the word *cuer*, heart, and that the translation is 'more at heart' (Webster's Third International Dictionary). This might lead us to think of titles such as *Lionheart* and *Braveheart* and to contemplate exemplary courage and heroism. Moral courage appears as a central virtue in the work of most, if not all, key virtue theorists (see the lists of virtues in the Appendix). Comte-Sponville (2002, p. 44), for example, writes:

> Of all the virtues, courage is no doubt the most universally admired. What is unusual is that the prestige it enjoys seems not to depend on the society, the period, or even, for the most part, the individual. Cowardice is everywhere despised and bravery everywhere esteemed.

One of the earliest and best-known accounts is by Aristotle (1976 edition, 1115a6–29) who described courage as 'the right attitude towards feelings of fear and confidence' and 'a mean state in relation to feelings of fear and confidence'. Courage, on this account, requires a certain attitude towards fear and confidence. To be courageous, people need to strive towards what Aristotle called a mean (see Chapter 3) and, therefore, to avoid an excess (foolhardiness or over-confidence) and a deficiency (cowardice or deficient confidence). He goes on to say:

> undaunted, so far as is humanly possible, he [sic] will fear what is natural to fear, but he will face it in the right way and as principle directs, for the sake of what is right and honourable [...] the man who faces and fears (or similarly feels confident about) the right things for the right reason and in the right way is courageous.
>
> (Aristotle, 1976, 1115a30-b19)

Hursthouse (1999, p. 115) points out that the 'wrong amount' (and 'wrong occasion') relates to whether the object in question is appropriate. She reminds us that the things which it is natural to fear, according to Aristotle, are 'death, great pain and fairly extensive damage' (p. 114). She suggests that:

> fearing the right things the right or wrong amount is fearing them somewhere between too much and too little. What fearing death 'the right amount' comes to is fearing death the right way, and what that comes to is fearing an ignoble dishonourable death but not fearing an honourable one. And the same, I think, applies to fearing great pain and damage 'the right amount'.

Knowing what is the right thing to fear and how much to fear appears challenging. However, this is not, in our view, a weakness of a virtue-based ethics. Virtue ethics, as Hursthouse (p. 60) says, does not aim to produce an algorithm for life or for specific situations and people of good character are often the 'first to recognise that they do not know what ought to be done' (p. 62). Ethical aspects of life generally, and professional life in particular, are challenging and there is often uncertainty about the right object, what it means to be virtuous and to do the right thing in particular situations. What keeps the moral virtues on the ethical rails, as it were, is wisdom (examined in Chapter 4). The wise professional is able to perceive the salient aspects of a situation, to deliberate and to act.

We suggest in Chapter 1 that vulnerability is part and parcel of the human condition. Recognising the fears that service users and professionals experience goes some way towards understanding their vulnerability. Courage is arguably a response to human vulnerability but it need not deny dependence on others. Just as there are different types of vulnerability so there are different fears and different types of courage. It seems plausible to us that there is a correlation between types of vulnerability and types of courage, that is, physical, psychological, emotional, existential, social and moral. Fears that reinforce physical vulnerability might include fear of injury, illness or disease. Fears related to psychological and emotional vulnerability might include fears of irrationality, loss of control or confidence, or humiliation. Fears related to existential vulnerability could include fears of nihilism, meaninglessness or despair. Social vulnerability might be characterised in terms of fear of loneliness or isolation whereas moral vulnerability could relate to shame and disgust.

Courage can be characterised, in relation to different types of fears, as physical, psychological, emotional, existential, social and moral.

Particular situations may call for more than one type of courage and not all types will be moral. Pellegrino and Thomasma (1993, p. 109), for example, describe *physical courage* as relating to the work of firefighters or the exploits of Evil Knievel (a 'daredevil' motorcyclist who engaged in increasingly dangerous stunts) who risk (or risked) physical injury in the course of their activities. They distinguish this from *moral courage* which they refer to as 'fortitude'.

These types of courage are not mutually exclusive. The work of firefighters engaged in rescuing people from burning buildings is an example of physical courage that may be moral, that is, directed towards a good end. The firefighters are effectively *being for the good*. We do not agree that fortitude can be taken as synonymous with moral courage for two reasons. First, fortitude is not necessarily moral in that it may not be directed towards the good. We might, for example, imagine a mountaineer ascending Mount Everest in adverse conditions, enduring pain and confronting a range of fears, purely for self-serving and competitive reasons. We are not saying that mountaineering may not be directed towards moral ends but merely that it is not necessarily so. The mountaineer may be climbing Everest to raise money for a worthwhile charity. Physical courage and fortitude may, therefore, be described as moral or non-moral in the sense of being directed towards moral or non-moral ends.

Secondly, as with other virtues discussed in this text, courage as a virtue is a character trait comprising a 'complex network of dispositions' (Goldie, 2000, p. 157) and necessary to respond to the subtleties and complexities of fear-inducing situations. The aspiration to be courageous overall, to have courage as a composite virtue, is important. However, it is more likely that people demonstrate modules of courage. Adams (2006, p. 128) writes of 'modules forming a more inclusive composite disposition'. The modules may relate to different types of courage, to specific domains, to different dispositions to think, feel and act. So, for example, a professional might be physically courageous (ready to intervene should a service user become aggressive) but not psychologically or emotionally courageous (unable to break bad news to a service user perhaps). She may be courageous in her professional life but not in her private life. She may be courageous within her own professional group but less courageous in an inter-professional context. She may be disposed to endure hardship but not to speak out about unacceptable practice. She may, therefore, demonstrate behavioural dispositions such as the ability to work with limited resources or remain alongside service users when they are distressed or in pain (perhaps to be with someone who is grieving or a woman who is giving birth) but be unable to blow the whistle on bad practice.

For our purposes here, the distinction between moral and non-moral courage is particularly important. Sport and risk-taking activities such as mountaineering or bungee-jumping may, on the one hand, be described as non-moral albeit requiring physical, psychological and emotional courage. When climbing, for example, one has to remain calm and confront fears of falling. This does not appear to have moral content. On the other hand, it can be argued that sport and leisure activities also have a moral dimension. Participants may engage in these activities in ways that impact on other humans, other species and the environment in positive and negative ways. Using time in this way may also mean that individuals are less conscientious in personal and professional roles. Alternatively, their learning from participation in sporting activities may enhance their personal and professional capacities. Engaging in such activities with colleagues may, for example, contribute to team building, and a stronger team in health and social care may contribute to the flourishing of service users and professionals. People may also gain as individuals as such activities may help develop courage transferable to other areas so this may, therefore, contribute to the development of the virtue.

In addition to moral and non-moral courage it is necessary to consider the possibility of courage that is directed towards bad ends, courage that might be thought of as *being for the bad*. Comte-Sponville (2002, p. 45) cites Voltaire as stating that 'courage is not a virtue, but a quality shared by blackguards and great men alike'. Examples of those who have risked their lives for crime or unjust wars and who lack other virtues and/or possess vices would appear to be examples of immoral courage. Health care examples of immoral courage might include the incompetent professional who overcomes fears to carry out an advanced procedure on a patient with a view to enhancing his or her career prospects rather than improving the well-being of the patient. Courage here is accompanied by vices of, perhaps, callousness, vanity and improper ambition. Our view is that while such examples of courage directed towards immoral ends might be described as courage or bravery, they cannot be described as exemplifying a moral virtue. Courage as a virtue is necessarily directed towards good ends, be they moral (contributing to flourishing) or non-moral (contributing to fitness, resilience and confidence, for example).

Thus far, we have discussed different types of courage (physical, psychological, emotional, social and existential) and made a distinction between moral and non-moral courage. We distinguished also between modular and composite courage. Hursthouse, writing of virtue more generally, says that 'we do accept, as a fact, that people are rarely all of a piece as far as their virtue is concerned, we also recognise that the virtues do form some sort of a unity' (1999, p. 153). *Composite courage* is when courage is integrated as one of a range of virtues and where people can be relied on to confront fear and to promote the flourishing of themselves and others.

Courage – a health and social care professional virtue

The vignettes presented at the beginning of this chapter suggest the importance of courage in everyday professional practice. Jeremy discusses the challenging nature of social work practice when he describes fear-inducing and uncertain situations. His story also points to the need to consider the relationship between self-regarding and other-regarding aspects of courage. If he does not knock loudly enough, he will not experience the anger and violence he fears; but he will not be responding adequately to concerns regarding the safety and well-being of children and others. If he does knock loudly enough and he gets a response from the family, he may be at the receiving end of their anger but may be able to make some assessment of the situation. Reports from inquiries relating to child deaths all too often highlight the non-intervention of professionals as a contributory factor (see, for example, Laming, 2003). It may be that Jeremy concludes that children are not at risk. It may also be that he concludes that they are at risk and his intervention results in their being taken to a place of safety.

Jeremy is perhaps aware of his physical vulnerability and may lack confidence that he can respond to such a situation competently. If he chooses not to knock this may be because he is motivated by self-interest rather than by the interests of those who may need his help, because he is overcome by fear (so may be considered cowardly) or because he does not have sufficient confidence and competence to deal appropriately with the situation that may arise. Acknowledging one's limitations and lack of competence also requires courage. Jeremy may knock loudly enough, get a response from the family and then mismanage the situation provoking an angry or violent reaction. In that case he may be acting in a rash or foolhardy way rather than with courage. For Jeremy to demonstrate courage appropriately in such situations requires a certain level of confidence and also competence, knowledge about risk and safeguarding children, insight into his own motivation and a commitment to aspire to the flourishing of others as well as himself. What he requires, first and foremost, is practical wisdom. This helps Jeremy to see and understand the salient features of the situation, to deliberate well and to make a judgement as to the most ethical and appropriate action. Jeremy may also benefit from talking the situation through with experienced colleagues and, if necessary, from being accompanied and supported as he makes the visit. Other virtues also seem relevant here, for example, patience, temperance, care and respect. Professional integrity is an important professional virtue that will help moderate self-interest in such situations.

Some aspects of the Lourdes Hospital Inquiry resonate with other situations where practitioners raised concerns about poor practice. In the early 1990s, for example, the British nurse Graham Pink went public about the neglect of patients he witnessed at Stepping Hill Hospital, Stockport. He wrote as follows in the *British Medical Journal*:

> It was a disgrace that these patients, who had served their families, their communities, and their countries throughout the Second World War should be neglected in so shameful a way. In their last days and hours our senior citizens deserve close, personal attention and loving care from sufficient nurses and assistants who have the time to carry out their work in a calm and dignified manner – not the noisy, stressful, and furious way we were often obliged to rush to get the work done. No one should die alone in hospital. But it happened so often and will happen again tonight.
>
> (Pink, 1994, p. 1702)

Pink also wrote about the cost of whistle-blowing. He was dismissed from his job for 'breach of confidentiality'. An industrial tribunal ruled that he had been unfairly dismissed.

In July 2001, the Bristol Royal Infirmary Inquiry report (Kennedy, 2001) stated that up to 35 babies, who had undergone heart surgery, had died unnecessarily at the hospital. One journalist wrote:

> The vast and long-awaited report lifts the lid on the arrogance, ambition and 'muddling through' at the hospital in the early 1990's where 'too much power was in too few hands' and a 'club

culture' existed which shut out young doctors like Stephen Bolsin, who tried to raise concerns about the death rates.

(Boseley, 2001)

Although the actions of consultant anaesthetist, Stephen Bolsin, who went public about the situation at Bristol, were vindicated in the report findings, he secured an employment contract in Australia before making his concerns public. Bolsin (2003, p. 294) writes that 'whistleblowing is an extremely unpleasant experience'. Both Pink and Bolsin have become known in Britain as high-profile whistle-blowers. What is common to both is the experience of negative treatment. What is also common to both, it seems, is courage. Both took a stand and spoke out when others remained silent. Both advocated for vulnerable patients.

Similar examples can be found in the social work field. Machin (1998) gives an account of her experience as a social worker in a secure hospital for mentally disordered offenders in England, her decision to give evidence to a public inquiry investigating allegations of patient abuse and her subsequent dismissal from her job. She speaks of her own beliefs as being important:

My social work practice was born within the radical model. My formal training confirmed my belief that the traditional social work models need to be challenged in the light of human experience and emotion, and that workers need to get alongside their clients in order to foster empowerment and counteract the effects of their disabling conditions of life. My efforts to understand the context of the social and economic conditions in which my clients existed did not distance me from feelings of warmth and compassion, or from painful emotions born from understanding the effects of poverty and deprivation.

(Machin, 1998, p. 118)

Machin specifically locates herself within the 'radical model' – working for change in social conditions – whilst also retaining compassion for the people with whom she is working. One of the slogans of the early feminist movement was, 'the personal is political'. Machin's comments are a reminder that the professional is also political, that is, as a person in a professional role we have a duty publicly to challenge inhuman, degrading, unjust and oppressive practices committed by fellow professionals. Briskman (2005), writing from an Australian perspective on the abusive and inhumane treatment of indigenous people and asylum seekers by services that are delivered by social workers, exemplifies a similar commitment to expose and challenge unjust policies and practices with which social workers are often complicit. This was achieved through undertaking research, writing newspaper articles and campaigning with others within and outside the university where she worked.

We know less about the experience of midwives at the Lourdes Hospital following the investigations and the departure of Dr Neary. In the Lourdes Hospital Inquiry we are reminded that no one died but a large number of women, some young, had hysterectomies unnecessarily. It is most likely, therefore, that these women would have had more children. In a sense lives were lost.[3] The inquiry raised an important question that also applies to the Stepping Hill and Bristol situations: Why did other people not raise concerns?

Speaking out against unethical and unacceptable activities is not easy. People require, for example, a robustness or resilience to weather the consequences of taking a moral stand as in the case of whistle-blowing. It has been pointed out by Hunt (cited by Dobson, 1998, p. 12) that:

> We now have plenty of evidence that whistle blowing affects health. When people are put under that kind of stress in highly charged atmospheres, it can cause all kinds of illness.

A good many references are made to qualities of character in the Lourdes Hospital Inquiry report. Nurses and midwives were, the report states, required to be obedient, respectful, loyal and unquestioning. It was not, therefore, that those involved lacked virtues but rather that they lacked some virtues or perhaps modules of some virtues. The virtues, it is suggested in the report, that they may have had (for example, obedience, loyalty and respectfulness) do have a place in health and social care but do not comprise the total repertoire of virtues. The midwives who raised concerns leading to the investigation might be said to have had, at least, some modules of courage.

As with the other vignettes, our comments can only be speculative and tentative, since we do not have a fuller narrative nor the perspective of all the people involved. It is interesting to note that

---

[3] This point was made by Paul Wainwright.

Dr Neary was described by some of his colleagues as caring, kind and hardworking and by others as rude, crude and opinionated. His fear of haemorrhage suggests perhaps the lack of and need for different types of courage: physical courage to maintain a steady hand when there was haemorrhage during surgery; psychological courage to withstand the stress of the situation and to hold steady not proceeding to hysterectomy; and moral courage to keep sight of the ends of ethical rather than defensive medical practice. Perhaps he also had some modules of courage in some domains but not, it seems, in the operating theatre when there was severe haemorrhage.

The third vignette relating to Susan, a paramedic, emphasises the emotional dimension of courage. She talks of holding it together and of, sometimes, going against protocol to provide parents with closure, so they could see and believe that everything had been done. In relation to Susan's narrative it is possible that, as two virtuous practitioners might respond to the same situation in a different way, there may be different views about what being for the good or being virtuous entails. Another practitioner might have taken the view that her action in carrying out a resuscitation procedure on an obviously dead child constituted deception[4] and dishonesty. The view might have been taken that the honest response was to inform the parent that the child was dead and to provide necessary support. Another person may, however, consider Susan's response the most courageous and compassionate response. There are obviously challenges in relating vignettes to the analysis of virtue concepts and in focusing on one rather than several virtues in relation to each vignette. However, it is our view that interrogating these vignettes has value in clarifying the role and implications of individual virtues.

Susan's perspective also suggests that people should not make assumptions about the kinds of situations that professionals consider fear-inducing. For some, it may indeed be severe injuries, loss of blood or amputations but for others it may be the fear of the death of a child or of not responding appropriately to a distraught relative.

It is the case that health and social care professionals require courage for the everyday as well as the exceptional. To guide that courage professionals require practical wisdom. As Comte-Sponville (2002, p. 31) states, 'Without prudence [practical wisdom], the other virtues are merely good intentions that pave the way to hell'. Given

---

[4] Daniel Sokol made this suggestion.

the wide range of fears that professionals have to confront in their professional lives, courage is not optional but rather necessary for people to function adequately as professionals.

Strategies for practice and professional education

Engaging with literature and humanities

Reading and reflecting on exemplars of courage enables professionals to consider what courage involves and how this relates to their own practice. Frankl's (2004) description of survival in Auschwitz and other concentration camps during the Second World War provides profound insights regarding courage and hope in the most harrowing of circumstances. In the course of reading and discussing Frankl's account, students and practitioners might consider the factors that enable people to maintain their dignity when circumstances have the potential to degrade and humiliate. Students and practitioners may also find Bauby's (1997) account, *The Diving-Bell and the Butterfly*, helpful in developing their understanding of the experience and courage of someone with 'locked-in syndrome'.

Recent books by Brown (2007a, b) discussing examples of everyday and exemplary courage provide insights regarding what it means to be courageous. Some of the examples relate specifically to health and social care professionals who appeared to demonstrate courage and persistence in achieving their ends. Students might be encouraged, for example, to read of the life and the character of nurse Edith Cavell, who was executed for her part in assisting British soldiers in Belgium during the First World War (Brown, 2007a, pp. 8–35). They might be asked to consider what might contribute to people continuing to be for the good when being so endangers them? In relation to Edith Cavell, students and practitioners might consider also the relationship between empathy, personal or professional ideals and feelings of loyalty towards those on one side of a conflict or war situation. Cavell's description of responses to the arrival of German troops in Brussels is as follows:

> We were divided between pity for these poor fellows, far from their country and their people suffering the weariness and fatigue of an arduous campaign, and hate of a cruel and vindictive foe, bringing

ruin and desolation on hundreds of happy homes and to a prosper-
ous and peaceful land. Some of the Belgians spoke to the invaders in
German, and found they were very vague as to their whereabouts,
and imagined they were already in Paris; they were surprised to be
speaking to Belgians and could not understand what quarrel they
had with them. I saw several of the men pick up little children and
give them chocolate or seat them on their horses.

(Brown, 2007a, p. 21)

In the course of this chapter, we have referred to reports (Harding
Clark, 2006; Kennedy, 2001; Laming, 2003) detailing individual
and institutional shortcomings resulting in harm and distress in
health and social care. This literature has the potential to help
students understand individual and institutional factors that
contribute to or diminish ethical practice. In discussing examples of courage there is the opportunity also to consider the role
of professional or practical wisdom, for example, in developing
moral perception and the moral imagination and responding to
challenging situations.

Reflection on self, others and practice

The importance of reflection on one's own practice, the practice of
others and of sharing reflections with others cannot be overstated.
The Lourdes Hospital Inquiry report, for example, suggests a lack
of self-scrutiny in relation to obstetric practice and a too-trusting
attitude towards other professionals. Professional supervision, peer
support and discussion, team meetings, clinical ethics committees
and action learning sets can all encourage this kind of reflection in
safe environments.

Habituation and role modelling

Habituation is considered a process that is part of moral education
whereby people develop good character. It involves practice and
repetition. This is not, however, an unreflective or decontextualised
activity, but rather one that occurs in response to real practice situations and involves criticality and a sense of pleasure in being ethical (Sherman, 1999). Practising in real life and rehearsing difficult
situations through role play are all vital in developing the courage
required for professional life.

Observing and talking with people who demonstrate courage in everyday practice also helps us to consider the nature and implications of courage. One of the greatest learning opportunities is to accompany a highly experienced practitioner whilst they accomplish a challenging or dangerous task, or face a situation where they have to confront their fears and anxieties. We could imagine a social work student undertaking a practice placement accompanying Jeremy, the social worker featured in the first vignette, to visit a family. Seeing how Jeremy approached this difficult job, watching how he spoke to the parents and talking to him afterwards about his own fear and how he handled it are all ways of beginning to develop courage in the student. We could imagine that after observing Jeremy on several occasions knocking on a family's door and initiating a visit, the student might then take the lead with Jeremy in the background.

This is an important strategy in promoting all of the virtues professionals need to approach situations like this critically. In addition to asking what type and degree of courage is required in such situations, professionals might also ask 'how did I do?' and ' how can I do better next time?' The development of the virtues has also been suggested as being most significant in resisting potentially corrupting influences (MacIntyre, 1985).

Institutional strategies

The reports referred to in this chapter relating to the investigation of unethical practices in health and social care examine individual and institutional dimensions of these situations. In addition to considering how and why individuals act or omit to act as they do, it is also crucial to consider the institutional context. The inquiries relating to the Bristol Royal Infirmary and the Lourdes Hospital point also to the nature of institutional cultures and systems. In addition to strategies to support the ethical practice of individual practitioners, consideration needs also to be given to leadership and the systems in place to investigate deficits in care.

The development of leaders who acknowledge human fallibility and vulnerability and who promote cultures that are understanding and supportive rather than defensive, complacent and blaming is essential. Organisational philosophies and mission statements that employees and service users have helped develop and can own go some way towards supporting moral climates within organisations. It has been argued that technological improvements in the way data regarding performance, critical incidents and errors, is collected and interpreted may help reduce errors and institutional failings (Bolsin *et al.*, 2005). Other strategies might include the implementation of systems of audit, transparency regarding institutional processes and statistics, regular and reflective team meetings and team-building exercises. Such strategies have the potential to support moral climates within organisations, to anticipate problems, respond to human fallibility and reduce the need for practitioners to have to blow the whistle on poor practice.

Concluding comments

Courage is an important professional virtue enabling practitioners to resist organisational and societal forces that compromise professional ideals. People are generally benefited by courage. Friends, family and service users are better off if professionals are courageous. If cowardice or rashness leads professionals to betray their friends, neglect their families or fail to intervene when service users are threatened, then it is clear that others will be harmed rather than benefited.

Contemporary professional practice requires that practitioners are able to reflect on and act in accordance with the requirements of courage. Identifying the salient features of the circumstances and aspiring to a good end enables the individuals to overcome their fear. Daloz Parks (1993, p. 182) in her writing about business ethics writes of courage as:

> when one is able to move beyond fear because one can see a more adequate and compelling truth than the truth of the danger and can act, therefore, in response to the truth beyond the fear.

Fully appreciating a service ideal, acknowledging one's own fears and aspiring to composite courage promotes the flourishing of service users and professionals. Professionals need to aspire to be more courageous, to develop composite courage, but they need at least some modules of courage to fulfil even minimally the values of their profession.

Chapter 10

Integrity

Introduction

Integrity is rather a different kind of virtue concept to the others we have discussed so far (such as courage or trustworthiness). It seems to refer to an overarching disposition or capacity that enables the moral agent to hold together and balance the other virtues – a characteristic of the holistic 'good professional' described in Chapter 3. In this sense, integrity might be regarded as a kind of moral competence or capacity that people use to make sense of their ideals and actions as a whole and to act accordingly. Indeed, 'integrity' literally means 'wholeness', and is often associated with coherence of beliefs and ideals, consistency and reliability of action and being thoroughly and wholeheartedly good. As with the other virtue concepts, the term integrity is used in a variety of different ways, with moral philosophers and other theorists offering different (and sometimes incompatible) accounts of what it is. So in this chapter we will spend some time examining alternative accounts of integrity as a concept, before examining how we might understand and promote integrity as a virtue in a professional context. We will look at different conceptions of integrity in professional life, including the distinction between seeing this as personal integrity (a wholehearted commitment to a set of values relevant to all aspects of life) transferred to a professional context; or as something distinctive (a wholehearted commitment to a set of professional values).

Vignettes

As a starting point, we will offer two vignettes relevant to the theme of integrity in professional life. The first is an account taken from a professional misconduct hearing about the dishonest actions of a nurse, which could be interpreted as damaging her integrity as a professional as well as the integrity of the profession of nursing.

The second vignette is drawn from an interview with a senior youth work practitioner working in a youth offending team and shows him struggling to preserve his integrity as a person and as a professional in a difficult organisational climate. Both practitioners left their jobs, but in the first case this was because the nurse had compromised her professional integrity and was removed from the register of professional practitioners; in the second case it was in order that the practitioner might preserve his personal and professional integrity.

1) The nurse who falsified data and was removed from the register

Sharon was a registered nurse employed by a national organisation to carry out interviews with members of the public as part of a five-year research project. The research was government funded and was intended to track health changes in 3500 people taking factors such as diet, occupation and the local environment into consideration. One of the participants in the research programme contacted the research organisation to say that the nurse had failed to keep an appointment with her to carry out an interview. On investigation, a completed interview form was found in respect of the participant. This raised concerns, so the nurse's interview records were checked and it was found that on six occasions she had claimed expenses for interviews she had not carried out and that she falsified the research data, including dates of birth and signatures on consent forms, in respect of six interviewees.

The research organisation referred the case to the Nursing and Midwifery Council Professional Conduct Committee, which investigated the allegations and held a hearing. The nurse did not attend the hearing, but had written to admit all the charges. The Committee decided to remove the nurse's name from the professional register. The NMC report of this case concludes that:

> The Chair said that her dishonesty was premeditated, recurrent and involved falsified consent, breach of trust, and theft. Her actions undermined trust and confidence in the professions and affected public perception of the research body and its findings.
> (Source: adapted from Nursing and Midwifery Council (NMC), 2004, pp. 12–13)

2) The youth offending team manager who quit

George qualified as a youth worker 22 years ago and had worked as a face-to-face practitioner, then as an area manager. When new multi-professional youth offending teams were set up in England to work with young offenders and undertake preventive work, he applied for the post of manager of a team covering a semi-rural area. The team comprised social workers, probation officers, community and youth workers, police, education welfare and health workers. George was in the post for about a year, before deciding to leave. He found it impossible to perform the job in the way he thought it should be done. The way George described his approach to his work suggested that he held a view of the goal of the social welfare professions as being about giving care and promoting welfare (in this case, young people's welfare) and doing this in a way that respected young people. Whilst he realised that there would always be imperfections and compromises, his experience in the youth offending team was very far removed from this conception of the professional caring role. He gave as an example the inability to provide adequate accommodation for young people who were remanded by the courts into the care of the local authority. The young people would often have to wait for hours on end whilst workers tried desperately to find a place for them to stay. Suitable accommodation for young people was scarce, of dubious quality and very expensive (requiring long negotiations with senior management in charge of children's and young people's services, which held the budget for this aspect of the work).

During the interview with George he commented, 'I couldn't be part of that, you know':

> In the end it was, it was getting to me so much, you know, that I had to kind of move for my own – for myself. Because it's – I think anybody who cares about people and who sees that, and who comes up against the brick walls, you know, on a daily basis, you can only take so much really, as one person.

He ended his account by saying that if he had not quit the job, 'I think it would have a lasting effect on my own self really'.
(Source: Individual interview)

Reflections

Sharon's case is described largely in terms of the actions of the nurse in question. Although the term 'professional integrity' is not mentioned in the summary of the case, we would suggest that Sharon's professional integrity was called into question by her actions. The falsification of the interviews, consent forms and travel claims amounted to dishonest behaviour and therefore compromised Sharon's role as a nurse. These actions are clearly in breach of the Nursing and Midwifery Council (2002) code of professional conduct that was in use at the time, which stipulates that registered practitioners must protect and support the health of patients and the wider community, act in such a way that justifies public trust and uphold and enhance the good reputation of the professions.[1] Submitting falsified data to a research project designed to benefit public health is contrary to the first point, whilst the dishonesty undermines trust in this nurse and the profession in general. The comments of the Chair of the hearing are particularly important, in that they draw attention to the fact that the dishonesty was premeditated and recurrent. This indicates that there are no mitigating circumstances to take into account that might reduce the seriousness of the offences, enable the nurse's integrity to remain more or less intact and therefore allow her name to remain on the register. Sharon herself did not appear at the hearing and there were no witnesses to testify that her behaviour was 'out of character', a single instance that could be recovered, or a mistake.

George did not mention the term 'integrity' in his interview either, nevertheless we can easily interpret his comments as justifying his leaving the job as a way of preserving his personal and professional integrity. He talks about the lasting effect on his 'own self' if he had stayed – implying potential damage, saying he 'couldn't be part of that'. This worker clearly had a view of what 'we' (social professionals) should be doing with young people in difficulty – which could be described as a kind of 'care'. Given that no matter how hard he tried he did not seem able to change the system, he left. It could be argued that by leaving he was abrogating his professional responsibility to change a flawed and damaging system. Yet given he felt he had hit 'brick walls', he felt justified in leaving to preserve himself

---

[1] A new code was introduced in 2008, expressing similar sentiments, although with some significant changes, which are discussed later in this chapter.

intact to take a more worthwhile job (in fact, he moved on into a senior management post in the community and youth work field).

In the vignette relating to Sharon's case, we do not have any account of her views and do not hear her voice. So judgement about the breach of professional integrity is based on the accounts given of her behaviour. George's case, on the contrary, shows a practitioner giving an account of his response to a difficult working environment, and attempting to justify his decision to get out of this situation by demonstrating how it did not allow him or others to function as 'good professionals' according to his ideal standard of good social care work. This is an example of a professional practitioner giving a performance as a person of integrity through his talk in the course of the interview, and shows how 'integrity' is created in the accounts that people give of themselves and their actions.

Before examining integrity in professional life in more detail, we will first explore the nature of integrity. If we regard integrity as an overarching virtue or moral quality that involves holding together the other virtues, then a person of integrity will both have the other virtues and be able to hold them in balance as a unified whole. Interpreted in this way, integrity has both a form (wholeness, consistency, balance) and content (virtues of honesty, truthfulness and so on). This is readily seen in George's case, where he seemed to be concerned about holding himself intact in relation to a set of values that included respect and care for young people. We will now offer a brief overview of several different accounts of the nature of integrity, some of which focus more on its form and others on its content.

Form: consistency and commitment[2]

We will outline briefly below two of the alternative accounts that have been given of integrity, which focus on consistency and coherence.

The integrated self

According to this view, integrity is a matter of people integrating various parts of their personality into a harmonious intact whole.

---

[2] Some of the material in this section of the chapter draws on article by Sarah Banks (2004), 'Professional integrity, social work and the ethics of distrust', *Social Work and Social Sciences Review*,' vol. 11, no. 2, pp. 20–35.

This entails the ordering of conflicting desires, commitments, principles and values and hence avoiding or resolving conflict (see Frankfurt, 1987 for a discussion of 'wholeheartedness' and the integrated self). Being 'wholehearted' in this sense involves prioritising desires or principles and acting on those that are judged as more worthwhile, for example, valuing healing the sick over making a profit or vice versa. Although there are many versions of what counts as a 'self', which we will not rehearse here, it is noteworthy that we do often talk of integrity in terms of the 'self'. In the second vignette, George spoke of his work having a lasting effect on his 'own self'. However, this integrated self version of integrity as intact personality is a purely formal account – that is, it focuses on the consistency and coherence of a person's desires, virtues, principles and so on, rather than on the normative content of those that are prioritised. In George's case, for example, it would ignore the fact that it was consistency of actions with the professional values of care and respect that was at stake. As Cox *et al.* (2005, p. 2) point out, this view of integrity could allow for a used car salesperson to be wholeheartedly committed to selling cars for as much money as possible, which might mean them being prepared to lie. They suggest that we would not normally use the term 'integrity' to describe such a person.

Identity

Another essentially formal view of integrity particularly associated with the philosopher Bernard Williams (1973, 1981) involves holding steadfastly true to certain identity-conferring commitments or ground projects. He argues that these 'commitments' are projects with which people are deeply and extensively involved and identified. Abandoning these projects would mean losing touch with what gives their lives an identity. Such commitments might include supporting a cause (for example, a political party or the abolition of chemical and biological warfare) or they may be projects that flow from a more general disposition such as hatred of injustice, cruelty or killing (Williams, 1973, p. 111). This involves people acting from motives, interests and commitments that are most deeply their own. Like the integrated self version of integrity, according to this account of integrity there are no normative constraints on what people's commitments might be or what the they might do in pursuit of them. It might lead us to describe Hitler, who steadfastly pursued his project to eliminate the Jews, as a person of integrity, for example. Furthermore, it does not take account of occasions when it would seem plausible to suggest that integrity might involve giving up one's commitments (changing course, realising we are following a flawed or bad project).

The criticisms of the integrated self and identity accounts of integrity amount to the fact that they fail to capture the substantive content of the desires, values, projects and commitments that are being held together or pursued. One way round this problem, which some commentators have adopted, is not to say that these are inadequate accounts of the generic concept 'integrity' but rather to distinguish between 'personal integrity' and 'moral integrity'. The term 'personal integrity' is used to characterise integrity that is mainly about consistency, while 'moral integrity' has a normative component. On such a view, Hitler could be characterised as a man of personal integrity, but not of moral integrity. For Cox *et al.*(2003, 2005), to call someone a person of integrity who holds to projects or has committed acts that are commonly judged evil or morally wrong is a misuse of the term 'integrity'. Such debates are largely academic, but it is important to note that 'integrity' is a complex concept, that is used in a variety of different ways along a continuum of form, content and agent commitment. In this chapter we do not use the distinction between moral and personal integrity as described above. We use the term 'integrity' in its moral sense, that is, to refer to persons and actions exhibiting the quality of moral wholeness. We use 'personal integrity' as a global concept to mean integrity across a person's life (as distinct from more localised concepts such as 'professional integrity').

Content: conduct and character

Much recent philosophical literature on integrity (for example, Calhoun, 1995; Cox *et al.*, 2003, 2005; Graham, 2001) is particularly critical of accounts of integrity that focus simply on its form. We will now consider other versions of integrity that focus more on the substantive content of what we value or are committed to, including accounts that describe integrity in terms of people's actions (conduct) and character traits (virtues).

Conduct according to socially accepted moral norms/standards

The term 'integrity' is often used loosely to refer to generally honest, trustworthy conduct. As Cox *et al.* (2005, p. 1) comment, sometimes it is used almost synonymously with 'moral' – that is, acting according to commonly held moral norms. This characterisation is most frequently found in ordinary usage or non-philosophical literature. It is also often used in the local context of integrity in certain professional or public offices or roles. Here primarily what counts is people's actual conduct, rather than their commitments or motivations, as in the case of Sharon, the nurse who falsified data. This version of integrity does include a normative element, but at the same time it omits the sense of strong ownership of the norms/standards that was present in the two versions noted earlier. If we are looking for a version of integrity that entails moral agents taking the norms (critically) on board as their own, then a focus simply on conduct misses out this element of critical reflection, motivation, commitment and ownership of values or 'regulative ideals' (which we find in George's account of his decision to quit his job).

Social virtue

One approach to integrity that goes further towards capturing both its form and its content is to see integrity as a social virtue. According to Calhoun (1995), integrity involves 'standing for something' that is personally endorsed by the moral agent, but this is in a social context that provides a broader reference point for evaluating the worth of the projects/commitments. Calhoun argues that persons of integrity do not just act consistently with what they personally endorse, they stand up for their best judgement within a community of people trying to discover what in life is worth doing. Integrity is a matter of having proper regard for one's role in a community process of deliberation over what is valuable and what is worth doing. This entails not only standing up, unhypocritically, for one's best judgement, but also that one has proper respect for the judgement of others. Cox *et al.* (2005, p. 6) argue that this version of integrity still has limitations in that having regard to 'what in life is worth doing' does not necessarily mean that the answers to that question will be moral or other-regarding.

Complex and thick virtue

Cox *et al.* (2003, 2005, p. 9) themselves suggest that the concept of integrity may be better conceived as a 'cluster concept' that lies together different overlapping qualities of character. They argue that integrity is a virtue, but it is more complex than many of the other virtues (such as courage or benevolence). Hence they characterise 'integrity' as a 'complex and thick virtue term'. They use the Aristotelian characterisation of virtue as a mean between two excesses (although Aristotle himself does not discuss integrity as a virtue in this way). They suggest that it stands between the qualities associated with inflexibility such as arrogance, rigidity, dogmatism, sanctimoniousness and those associated with superficiality and artificiality, such as capriciousness, weakness of will, self-deception, hypocrisy. The person of integrity, they suggest, 'lives in a fragile balance between every one of these all-too-human traits' (Cox *et al.*, 2003, p. 41). They argue for an account of integrity as 'a capacity to respond to change in one's values or circumstances, a kind of continual remaking of the self, as well as a capacity to balance responsibility for one's work and thought' (Cox *et al.*, 2003, p. 41). This is a much more dynamic account, which does not require a concept of an unchanging self or rigid identity. They also argue that there are normative restrictions on what a person of integrity may do, suggesting that attributions of integrity presuppose 'fundamental moral decency' (Cox *et al.*, 2003, p. 41). That is, people of integrity act on commitments that a reasonable person could accept as important (Cox *et al.*, 2003, p. 65). This, of course, leaves open for debate what is regarded as 'fundamental moral decency', but we can assume that the substantive content mentioned earlier (such as honesty, fairness, truth-telling) is what would count. This account of integrity as a virtue takes account of many features of our ordinary usage of the term, including the fact that it is about both wholeness (form) and soundness (moral content).

Process: moral competence

On the above account, to be a person of integrity entails having a capacity to do the work necessary to sustain one's fragile self. Cox *et al.* (2003) talk of the capacity to respond to change and a continual remaking of the self. This has resonances with Walker's (1998) characterisation of integrity as 'reliable accountability', requiring a kind of moral competence in resolving conflicts and priorities, readjusting ideals and compromising principles. This is part of Walker's 'expressive-collaborative' approach to ethics, which regards the story as the basic form of representation for moral problems (Walker, 1998, p. 110). Within this, integrity can be regarded as a kind of reliable accountability that we construct in the stories we tell about our relationships, identities and values. Stories are reworked and revised and help us to see 'sense-making connections [that] serve to bundle up varied or repeating actions into legible configurations, such as neglecting a friendship or trying to disown a past' (Walker, 1998, p. 110). Walker argues that the point of integrity is 'to maintain – or reestablish – our reliability in matters involving important commitments and goods' (Walker, 1998, p. 106). It is based on the assumption that human lives are changing and are deeply entangled with others. We are often seeking, therefore, a local dependability (rather than global wholeness) and a responsiveness to the moral costs of error and change rather than consistency.

The stories people tell may well be about integrating selves, maintaining identity, displaying qualities of character and conduct. This approach to integrity as a kind of moral competence usefully extends its characterisation as a thick and complex virtue and enables us more easily to undertake empirical explorations of integrity. It also links with MacIntyre's (1985) idea of the narrative unity of a life (see Chapter 2 for a discussion of MacIntyre's virtue ethics).

Integrity in professional life

If we regard our earlier discussion as being about 'personal integrity' or integrity in general, then what is 'professional integrity' or integrity in professional life? Do we just extrapolate and say it is personal integrity manifested in a work role? Or is it something distinctive? How we view professional integrity will depend upon our view of the relationship between the ethics of personal and professional life. We suggested earlier in the book that the ethical norms attaching to the role of being a professional health or social care worker are *not the same* as those to which we would adhere in everyday life (for example, it is not regarded as appropriate to develop a deep personal friendship with a patient/service user; professionals have special duties of confidentiality). Nevertheless they are a *development* of the values by which we would operate in everyday life – in particular, according to Koehn (1994, pp. 154 ff) an intensification of the relationship of trust.

Musschenga (2001) distinguishes between global and local concepts of integrity. The former refers to coherence and consistency between beliefs and values across all roles and domains of life, while the latter applies in a particular role or context. Examples given of local integrity include professional, occupational, civic, political and managerial. According to Musschenga, all local forms of integrity have substantive content (that is, they are not purely formal) given by the role context. Using this local–global distinction is useful in helping us examine the nature of professional integrity, which we suggest could be seen in at least two ways:

1. *Personal integrity in professional life* – a global concept (personal integrity) manifested in a local context (professional role).

2. *Professional-integrity* – a local concept referring to the general honesty and reliability of the person acting in that professional role. The hyphen has been used to distinguish this specific concept, 'professional-integrity' from the generic concept of 'professional integrity', which is often used also to include 'personal integrity in professional life'.

The distinction is quite a fine one, but just serves to place the focus in the first case on the *personal values* as manifested or indeed modified in the professional role and in the second case on the *professional values*, as developed and debated by a community of practitioners (albeit revised and accepted by the individual person taking on the role).

Personal integrity in professional life

The concept of 'personal integrity in professional life' could be seen as placing the emphasis on the unity of personal and professional life – seeing either no separation between the two (one simply acts with everyday honesty, reliability and so on in one's work role) or a strong continuity and connection (one has chosen the job as a vocation and actively strives to live up to one's personal values and projects through the job).

Acting in accordance with commonly accepted everyday ethical standards in professional life may seem to go without saying, yet there may be occasions when the demands of the job seem to offend against our normal standards of respect and decency. Keeping young people waiting for hours in an office whilst accommodation is found (as recounted by George in the second vignette) may be one example.

In George's case, however, his moral objection to the requirements of his job seems stronger than this. George presents himself as having a deep commitment to caring about people, which is presumably why he trained to be a youth worker. The term 'vocation' may be too strong to apply in this case, but certainly it has some resonances. We usually use the term 'vocation' when people actively choose a profession or occupation so that they can live out their personal moral values in and through their work (see Bellah *et al.*, 1988, p. 66; Blum, 1994, p. 104). An ideal version of this would be that there are no contradictions and conflicts (perhaps a Buddhist monk may come close to this). A more realistic version would be that the aim is to reconcile personal and professional values and roles as far as possible, which may involve recognition of the need for compromise and readjustment of both personal and professional values. Although regarding health or social care work as a vocation in an ideal sense may be relatively rare these days because of the organisational constraints in voluntary, private and statutory sector work, there is no doubt that many practitioners still hope for some congruence between their personal values and those embodied in the work they do. Indeed, Hoggett *et al.* (2006) note the strong sense of emotional commitment that people working in the public services bring to their jobs, showing in their study of regeneration workers how such professionals are often motivated by a 'reparative impulse' (a passionate desire to undo some of the damage that has been done to others). Certainly, the ideal of 'vocation' may still be used as a yardstick against which to measure 'how bad things have got' and in deciding when to change jobs (as in George's case) or 'blow the whistle' (as in the case of the various practitioners discussed in Chapter 9 in relation to courage).

Professional-integrity

The concept of 'professional-integrity' focuses on how the person in the role matches up to and holds on to the values of the profession. This may be looked at in two ways, which, following Cox *et al.* (2003) can usefully be distinguished as 'professionalism' and 'ideal professional integrity'. Professionalism entails holding on to the extant values of the profession as outlined in a professional code and accepted by the current community of practitioners (as in the case of Sharon given earlier, who failed to practise in accordance with the professional values in the NMC code). Ideal professional integrity involves holding on to a more timeless service ideal of what the profession should be at its best (as seems to be the case with George).

In the case of Sharon, as noted earlier, her actions were judged in relation to the standards in the NMC (2002) code of conduct that was current at the time. Although that particular code does not use the term 'integrity', the latest version (NMC, 2008) does include 'integrity' as part of what is required for public trust in nurses and midwives who should

> work with others to protect and promote the health and wellbeing of those in your care, their families and carers, and the wider community; provide a high standard of practice and care at all times; be open and honest, act with integrity and uphold the reputation of your profession.
>
> (NMC, 2008)

Many other codes of ethics also include integrity as a key value (for example, Australian Association of Social Workers, 1999; British Association of Social Workers, 2002; National Association of Social Workers, 1999). The statement produced by the National Association of Social Workers in the USA sums up integrity as follows:

> Social workers are continually aware of the profession's mission, values, ethical principles, and ethical standards and practice in a manner consistent with them. Social workers act honestly and responsibly and promote ethical practices on the part of the organizations with which they are affiliated.

The focus is on the *actions* of the social worker *as a professional*. This statement suggests that professionals need to be aware of the totality of the aims, values, rules and so on of the profession as a whole and ensure that their actions are consistent with these norms. That is, they must see the profession as a coherent whole and their behaviour must fit within this professional framework. This particular statement implies that the professional framework is given and social workers need to be aware of it all the time. It does not present social workers as actively owning, reflecting on, questioning or contributing to the development and revision of the profession's values. This does not mean that this does not happen, that it is not valued, or that the importance of reflection does not appear elsewhere in the NASW code, just that this is not part of the description of 'integrity' given in the NASW code. In addition to acting in accordance with the specific normative content of the professional ethical framework, social workers are said to act honestly and responsibly. As noted earlier, honesty is a quality frequently associated with integrity. The British Association of Social Workers' code (BASW, 2002, para 3.4.2) elaborates a set of principles under the heading of integrity, which includes social workers being honest about their qualifications and competence, not using professional relationships for personal gain and not engaging in intimate or sexual conduct with service users.

What we call 'ideal professional integrity' is somewhat stronger than professionalism in that it goes beyond what the professional codes and guidance currently promote. It entails holding true to the goals or service ideals of the profession. We discussed service ideals in Chapter 1. Although problematic if we wish to designate service ideals as 'internal goods' located within identifiable professions, we suggested in Chapter 1 that the concept does perform a useful function as a 'regulative' or guiding ideal for individual practitioners. The notion of 'service ideal' encompasses both the idea of giving for the public good ('service') and a semi-transcendent value or aspiration ('ideal') (see Banks, 2004, pp. 53–58 for a fuller discussion of service ideals). Examples of service ideals include 'health' for medicine, and 'welfare' for social work (Airaksinen, 1994; Koehn, 1994; Oakley and Cocking, 2001). This is probably what Cox *et al.* (2003, p. 103) mean when they refer to the pursuit of a 'semi-independent ideal of what the profession should be at its best'. Pursuit of such an ideal might lead a professional practitioner to stand firm against their employer or indeed the professional association's current principles because they conflict with what is judged to be the broad goal of the profession. This is the account of professional integrity perhaps most commonly encountered in the literature of professional ethics (for example, Oakley and Cocking, 2001, pp. 82–83). However, it may be less easy to achieve in practice if the notion of discrete professions with commonly recognised service ideals is disintegrating as noted in Chapter 1. Clearly George, in addition to his concern with preserving his personal integrity ('my own self'), was also concerned to hold onto his ideal of the core purpose of the social welfare professions – that is, the promotion of social welfare in a caring and respectful manner.

Key elements of integrity in professional life

It will be noted that we have suggested that the case of George might be interpreted as exhibiting elements of both the global (personal integrity in professional life) and the local (professional-integrity) conceptions of integrity. This highlights the number of different strands that are part of the concept of integrity in professional life, which may overlap and are not mutually exclusive. Our depiction of the different versions of integrity in professional life suggests that integrity entails that professionals exhibit the following characteristics:

▶ *A commitment to a set of values*, the content of which relates to what it means to be a 'good person in a professional role' and/or a 'good professional'. In virtue ethical terms, this might include a regulative ideal of what kind of person an excellent professional practitioner would be.

▶ *An awareness that the values are inter-related to each other and form a coherent whole* and that their inter-relationship is what constitutes the overarching goals or purpose of the profession. This requires the perceptual and cognitive qualities associated with professional wisdom.

▶ A *capacity to make sense of professional values* and their relationship to a practitioner's own personally held values. This also requires professional wisdom – particularly the ability to reason and reflect.

▶ *The ability to give a coherent account* of beliefs and actions. This requires both practical skill in communication and an intellectual understanding.

▶ *Dispositions to think, feel and act in accordance with the core values.* This is about the professional cultivating all the virtues through professional practice and education.

▶ *Strength of purpose and the ability to implement these values.* This requires courage and determination.

Strategies for practice and professional education

If these are the key elements of integrity in professional life, then what do we need to do to foster and promote this 'thick and complex [social] virtue'? We make a number of suggestions below.

Developing, debating and owning professional values

If commitment to a set of values lies at the heart of integrity in professional life, then it is clearly important in professional education to discuss, debate, refine and develop a sense of ownership of the professional values as stated in the codes and other professional literature. Professional values are often presented in the form of very generalised lists of statements of principles or moral qualities, externally created and de-contextualised. To develop commitment to the values entails questioning and interpreting them, and above all, exercising critical reflection and reflexivity during the course of practitioners' own work. Sharing experiences with colleagues or supervisors can help this process, as can studying case examples and vignettes and working through dilemmas and problems. Dilemmas by definition involve choosing between alternative courses of action where the right one is not clear. To attempt to resolve a dilemma involves a process of weighing up and balancing values, priorities and consequences. Encouraging students in professional education and practitioners in supervision and continuing professional development to undertake a process of consciously asking themselves how their actions cohere with their own values and those of the profession can be a useful exercise.

Awareness of and location within a professional tradition

A sense of the history of the profession or occupational group to which a practitioner belongs, its changing roles and values, is also important in locating the current roles and values in a context, and reminding us that these are constantly subject to change and revision. 'What is good practice?' and 'What kind of person is a good professional?' are questions that stimulate us to think about the profession or occupational group as a whole, how what counts as 'good' may have changed and is the subject of ongoing debate, especially in inter-professional contexts. Often professionals bemoan changes that have taken place in their work settings, looking back to a time in the past when conditions were 'better' and trying to hold on to this vision. Yet if they are to remain in jobs and preserve integrity, they may have to adjust their ideals to new circumstances as well as try to change aspects of the new context that are inimical to 'good practice'.

Practising dialogue and debate

If a large part of performing as a person professional integrity entails a process of reflexive sense-making and the giving of coherent accounts, then it is also important that practitioners develop the capacity to be reflexive and to talk of themselves and their work in ways that are plausible and credible to themselves, colleagues, employers, other professionals and the wider public. Hence practising the giving of accounts, entering into debate and dialogue as students and professionals in the context of their peers is an important set of skills to learn and rehearse. Pithouse and Atkinson (1988) speak of the 'ethnopoetics' of professional talk (referring particularly to social work). The term 'ethnopoetics' is usually used to refer to the oral telling of native stories and myths, for example, those of native American peoples (see Hymes, 1981; Sammons and Sherzer, 2000), which have an internally recognised form (certain kinds of language, style, repetitions and so on). While it may be stretching the analogy somewhat to apply the concept to everyday talk amongst professionals in a literate culture, there is no doubt that part of what 'being a good professional' entails is the ability to give a competent performance as 'good professional' (Taylor and White, 2000; White and Stancombe, 2003).

Being part of and working through professional groups and networks

We noted that integrity is often invoked in situations of adversity – when someone's values are undermined or threatened. This means practitioners need courage to stand up for their beliefs and act in accordance with them. They may need to resist pressures to cover up or conform, as shown in the cases of the various whistle-blowers described in Chapter 9. Solidarity with other work colleagues and through professional associations, political networks and trade unions is also important in such cases. Individual practitioners, no matter how resilient or courageous, risk victimisation and disempowerment if they stand alone as isolated individuals.

Concluding comments

We have suggested that 'integrity' can be understood in a number of different ways, but overall it covers the way in which people make sense of the values, relationships and commitments that are parts of their lives and work. Integrity in professional life, or professional integrity, is often regarded as the same as 'professionalism' and is invoked when professionals infringe professional standards (as in the case of Sharon) and hence their professional integrity is called into question. We find it equally interesting to consider cases where people attempt to maintain professional integrity in hostile organisational climates (as in the case of George). George gave an account of how he attempted to hold onto a particular vision of a society and of a profession, a set of values and principles judged to be important and a view of himself as a 'good practitioner' in circumstances that might be described as at best indifferent and were often hostile to his visions and values.

This suggests that practitioners need a capacity to make sense of how they act in a work role in the context of a broader narrative of ideals, values, character and consistency. Having a capacity and the moral competence to do this is important, so that practitioners working with vulnerable people can play a role in challenging systems of which the procedures and outcomes often perpetuate and encourage injustice, disrespectful treatment and a lack of genuine care and sensitivity. 'Integrity', as this process of reflexive sense-making, is part of what contributes to people's capacity to 'blow the whistle' on bad practice, to protest against injustice and to challenge demeaning behaviour. It is part of contributing to the development of better practice and a constant process of revision of accepted professional values and commitments in the light of new challenges and demands. If practitioners are to be able to remain in their jobs and maintain professional integrity, rather than quit jobs in order to preserve their professional integrity (as in the case of George), then they require not just a commitment to a set of professional values (as articulated in professional codes) but courage, commitment and a sense of solidarity. Professional integrity is very important in current health and social care practice, particularly if it can be used as part of an active ethics of resistance, which not only maintains commitment to a set of professional values and ideals, but also serves to promote their critical re-examination and recreation.

Chapter 11

Situating virtues in professional life

Introduction

In the early part of the book (Chapters 1 3) we outlined some features of a virtue-based approach to ethics, suggesting the relevance of this to the study and practice of professional ethics. We considered some criticisms and limitations of virtue ethics and outlined our own approach. We proposed that a virtue-based approach could usefully be regarded as one element in the understanding and practice of ethics in professional life. A virtue-based approach is a welcome complement to approaches or theories that tend to focus on the articulation and 'application' of principles and rules of professional conduct. It shifts the emphasis from principles, conduct and action to include other important features of ethics in professional life, namely, the professional practitioner or moral agent. Virtue ethics invites us to consider the person who perceives salient features of situations; who thinks, feels and acts in accord with dispositions; and who has motives, aspirations, ideals and emotions.

In Chapters 4–10 we explored the nature of relevant virtues (from professional wisdom to integrity) in the context of professional practice. These chapters gave examples of practitioners and service users deploying virtue concepts explicitly or implicitly in accounts of their work and experiences. We explored the nature of these concepts in the light of relevant moral philosophical and professional literature and considered what strategies might help promote these virtues in professional practitioners.

In this brief concluding chapter, we will reflect on the materials and arguments offered in the chapters on the specific virtues, attempting to pull together some general conclusions about the value and limitations of a virtue-based approach to ethics in professional life. First we will reflect and comment on the implications of the focus in virtue ethics on the dispositions of individual moral agents and how these relate to situational or organisational factors. We will then discuss the role of the virtues in a pluralist approach to ethics in professional life. Finally, we will consider how our approach fits in the developing trend towards inter-professional and integrated working in health and social care.

The individual moral agent in an organisational and political context

The vignettes at the start of each chapter featured accounts of practice, details of practitioners' roles and reflections by practitioners and others on their actions and roles. We used these accounts to shed light on the nature of practitioners' moral qualities or dispositions. For the most part, our focus has been on the individual practitioners, what kinds of people they are and how individual virtues can be developed through practice and professional education. One of the dangers of this focus is that it tends to pay less attention to the political and organisational context in which the work takes place. It may encourage us to regard the individual practitioner as personally responsible or blameworthy for the ethical failings of organisations, systems and institutions. Hardingham (2004) quotes empirical research undertaken by Chambliss (1996) in the United States into nurses' moral lives, which suggests that many of nursing's ethical problems are due to features of the systems in which they work, rather than individual moral failings:

> Remove a nurse with an ethical problem from the hospital, replace her, and her replacement will encounter the same problem. The problem is not of the person but of the system.
> (Chambliss, 1996, p. 91, quoted in Hardingham, 2004, p. 130)

Hardingham (2004, p. 130) interprets this research as suggesting that nurses face practical difficulties of 'accomplishing some task over the opposition of other people. They say, "I know what ought to be done, but I can't get it done"'. This leads her to claim that:

> Because the great problems of health care are structural and not the result of poor reasoning, the solutions cannot be created by

increasing education, holding ethics seminars, or (alas) writing books.

(Hardingham, 2004, p. 130)

The implication of this kind of argument is that it is difficult for individuals to change problems identified as 'structural' or 'systematic'. Certainly it is not easy, as evidenced by the youth justice team manager in the last chapter who quit his job because he was unable to improve the quality of services given to young people or treat them in ways that were respectful. Following Hardingham, we might say that he knew what ought to be done (provide good quality accommodation for young people quickly), but felt unable to do it. Hardingham suggests that these kinds of situations cause practitioners to feel 'moral distress'. This may in turn cause further moral suffering, negative emotions, self-doubt and self-blame (McCarthy and Deady, 2008, p. 257) and burnout (Sundin-Huard and Fahy, 1999). Such a vicious cycle makes tackling institutionalised constraints, poor or bad practice very difficult for individuals. Nevertheless, it can be done, as our account of the situation at the Lourdes hospital (Harding Clark, 2006) in Chapter 9 suggests. Here, despite structural and systemic problems, a few individuals, perhaps with the help of internal and external resources, challenged and put a stop to unethical practices.

Rossiter *et al.* (2000), in their empirical research on social workers' lived experience of professional ethics in Canada, identify similar issues to those raised by Hardingham and Chambliss, but construe them differently. They conclude that we should regard individual practitioners as having a significant role in both creating and responding to institutional systems and cultures. Rossiter *et al.* found social workers named the hierarchical and paternalistic nature of their organisations' management as 'agency politics'. As such they assumed far less responsibility for politics than they would for the resolution of ethical dilemmas. So, in effect, they were conceiving of their work situations in the way Hardingham describes – as constrained by institutional systems over which they had little or no control and that they had no power to change. Rossiter *et al.* (2000) interpret this as amounting to a separation of ethics from politics, and suggest this is not a productive way of looking at ethics. For 'agency politics' and systems of management are part of the process that conditions practitioners' perception of ethics:

Individuals are not 'susceptible' to organisations – they are constantly engaged, within mutually constituting relations with their organisations, in the business of making and being made as ethicists.

(Rossiter *et al.*, 2000, p. 91)

In other words, 'professional ethics' can be regarded as a discourse that is created and enacted through social relations. Organisational systems and structures create boundaries for ethical being and acting, while at the same time they are themselves created by people's ethical being and acting. This view of ethics and politics as intimately inter-twined would entail that individual practitioners should see them-selves as both formed by and forming the organisations for which they work, and as needing to engage in the critical tension this pro-duces. A recent survey by the Royal College of Nursing (2008) explor-ing nurses' views of dignity in care supports the view that we need to work at the level of politics, organisations and individuals to achieve changes in the ethics of professionals and ethos of organisations. Factors with the potential to maintain and diminish dignity in care were identified as: macro-level factors (for example, government poli-cies that support dignity in care and government waiting time targets that may compromise dignity); meso-level factors (for example, the provision or non-provision of adequate staff and material resources); and micro-level factors (the attitudes and behaviour of staff).

Some literature speaks of organisations as having a character (see Reiser, 1994). Whilst we do not tend to regard the character of an organisation in the same way as the character of individuals, people commonly do speak of the character of an organisation or group, meaning it has certain characteristic features relating to its ethos and culture. We might talk of a 'caring organisation' and by this we might mean: an organisation in which being caring is valued, promoted and even required in its staff. Such an organisation would have systems and ways of working that facilitate and require a car-ing approach; it would have staff members who are caring; and its culture and ethos would be caring (demonstrated in a range of ways, from the configuration of chairs in the waiting room to the attentive-ness of the receptionist). The character or moral qualities of people who work there and who sit on committees that manage and sup-port the organisation, along with the policies and procedures that guide the work, would all contribute to this organisational ethos. The term 'learning organisation' is used in a similar way, where people at every level are committed to work together to generate results they care about and desire (Senge, 2006).

Whilst some aspects of the character of organisations are difficult to change – especially those that are furthest away from the powers and influence of individual practitioners – it is important that practitioners have a critical awareness and understanding of the policies, procedures and other features of global, national and local cultures and economies that shape the characteristics and practice of the organisations and teams in which they work. Arguably what we have called the virtue of 'professional wisdom' embraces a critically reflective and reflexive mode of being. This entails an orientation to the work based on commitment to ideals of health, social welfare and social justice; an ability to engage in critical theorising about the current political context (including the use and abuse of power, the persistence of social and economic inequality and the oppression of marginalised groups in society); an awareness that things could be other than they are; and a commitment and ability to take action for change (Butcher *et al.*, 2007).

Many of the practitioners featured in our vignettes demonstrate this kind of critical awareness and commitment. Part of being ethical for them is engaging with situational and organisational constraints and seeing themselves as active moral agents who have some power to introduce change, although often at the micro-level of individual practice rather than the organisational or macro-political level. The accounts given in the vignettes in Chapters 4–10 make a good deal of reference to challenging circumstances in which practitioners report that they had inadequate resources to meet the needs of service users, found themselves in organisational cultures that did not prioritise individualised care or found it difficult to speak out about poor practice. In Chapter 6 (Respectfulness) the nurse-researcher, Ming-Li, discusses her experience of working in an institutional culture she considered disrespectful and dehumanising towards people with learning disabilities. In Chapter 9 (Courage), extracts from the *Lourdes Hospital Inquiry Report* (Harding Clark, 2006) reveal a complex interaction between individual and organisational ethical failings and the difficulties faced by a group of midwives in speaking out about the bad practice of a consultant obstetrician and gynaecologist. In Chapter 8 (Justice), a paediatric nurse, Lynne, talks about the challenge of allocating scarce resources and the need to fight a case for the value of a child being cared for at home. In the same chapter a social worker, James, discusses the difficulty of finding appropriate resources for people from minority ethnic groups with complex needs, suggesting the situation is discriminatory.

The vignettes suggest how we might conceptualise practitioners' responses to some of these very challenging circumstances in terms of particular moral dispositions or virtues. In Chapter 5 (Care), a student nurse describes how a qualified nurse was caring towards a patient during an uncomfortable procedure. A social worker (Debbie) in Chapter 6 gives an account of how she demonstrates respectfulness in advocating for a service user. In Chapter 9, a paramedic talks about 'mustering up courage' to maintain her professionalism and to prevent her from falling apart when dealing with the deaths of children.

Despite the focus on individual virtues, it is not our view that a virtue-based approach need privilege or prioritise individual dispositions or virtues over situational and broader political influences on ethical action. Rather we have argued for a two-pronged approach. In any given health or social care episode, the individual dispositions of the professional and the features of the situation, organisation and broader policy and political context are relevant to good actions and to being for the good. What we are proposing is, therefore, a situated virtue-based ethics, a professional ethics that addresses the character of individuals, groups, organisations and societies.

Webster and Baylis (2000), Hardingham (2004) and Ray (2006) point to the need to develop a moral community within organisations. Webster and Baylis (2000, p. 228) define this in a health context as 'a community in which there is coherence between what a healthcare organization publicly professes to be, and what employees, patients and others both witness and participate in'. It seems possible that the values of such an organisation (be they in health, social care or institutions providing professional education) will be influenced by the ethical expectations of employees, students, service users and others. Just as we specified the virtues relating to good character of individuals, it also seems helpful to specify these for organisations. Reiser (1994, p. 28) suggests that 'institutions, like their individual members, have ethical lives and characters' and that organisations need to demonstrate values such as humaneness, trust, fairness and dignity. It is possible, arguably, for a virtue-based ethics to apply to individual professionals and to the organisations to which they are affiliated. We need institutional structures and cultures that support the development of good dispositions or virtues in employees, board members and volunteers, who in turn contribute to and develop good organisations.

Virtues in context

Although we argued in Chapter 2 for a pluralist approach to ethical theory (that is, we do not favour the espousing of one single all-embracing theory that captures the whole of ethical life), in this book we have focused on presenting a virtue-based approach to ethics. A common challenge to a virtue-based approach is that it does not tell us what to do. Campbell (2005) refers to this as a problem of applicability. In fact, it is probably no more difficult to 'apply' virtue ethics in practice than it is to apply a principle-based ethical theory. It is a question of learning through experience, which takes time and effort. Hursthouse (1987, p. 247) suggests that it is a question of modelling ourselves on the 'fully virtuous person':

> The fully virtuous person, with full wisdom, would be the person who *knew* what to do or think in exactly those circumstances that many of us find so deeply puzzling [...] If the fully virtuous is described that way, it becomes clear that she is an ideal. We go for guidance to, or try to model ourselves on, the people who approximate to that ideal. Insofar as each of them fails to attain it, some will be better exemplars of certain virtues than of others.

Hursthouse is suggesting that the fully virtuous person would know what to do and think. If we want to know what to do, we model ourselves on such a person or go to her for advice. Of course, recognising the fully virtuous person is not so straightforward and, arguably, requires a good deal of wisdom learned in the context of a community of practitioners. The ability to recognise and emulate role models is, therefore, an important part of professional education and development.

What is often overlooked is that action guidance is not as forthcoming from other theoretical approaches to ethics as people might be led or like to believe. If we take a principle-based approach to ethics (as offered by Beauchamp and Childress, 2001), the principle to respect autonomy, for example, needs to be interpreted and considered in relation to specific circumstances and balanced with other principles. There is no principle or duty that is sufficiently clear to tell people exactly what to do in particular situations. Each situation is different as is each individual person. Professionals need to be sensitive to this. Just as a virtue-based approach may be complemented by a principle-based approach, so the latter also requires the virtues to respond to the particularities of individual situations. Professional wisdom is required for action based on principles just as it is for the moral virtues.

It is interesting to note that Beauchamp and Childress, often held up as the major exponents of principlism in professional ethics, introduced a whole chapter relating to virtues in professional life into the fourth edition of their textbook on biomedical ethics, acknowledging that:

> Principles require judgement, which in turn depends on character, moral discernment, and a person's sense of responsibility and accountability ... Often what counts most in the moral life is not consistent adherence to principles and rules, but reliable character, moral good sense, and emotional responsiveness.
>
> (Beauchamp and Childress, 1994, p. 462)

In the fifth edition of their book (Beauchamp and Childress, 2001), this chapter, renamed 'moral character', comes as a precursor to the coverage of principles.

As already mentioned, we espouse a position of ethical pluralism, meaning that we do not think that a single all-embracing theory based on one feature of ethical life (such as virtue ethics, Kantian duty-based ethics or utilitarianism) can encapsulate the whole of ethics. Any theoretical approach to ethics needs to include the virtues and relationships of individual moral actors, as well as impartial principles based on our duties to respect the rights of others and on the promotion of human welfare. At times, perhaps when working with challenging colleagues or service users, professionals may not always be able to think, act and feel in accord with the virtues and may need rules derived from principles or rights. As outlined in Chapter 2, important elements of professional ethics include:

- The character of the moral agent (the main focus of virtue ethics);
- The nature of right action (the main focus of deontological ethics);
- The outcomes of action (the main focus of consequentialist ethics);
- The relationships between people (the main focus of the ethics of care and proximity).

Inter-professional working in health and social care

We note at the beginning of the book the growing trend towards integrated services and inter-professional working across a range of professions concerned with the health and well-being of young people, families, vulnerable adults, neighbourhoods and communities. This in itself creates some ethical tensions as professions and professionals with particular sets of values, codes of ethics, professional cultures and organisational systems have to find ways of working together more closely in services, projects and teams. There is a growing literature describing and analysing some of the ethical issues and tensions that arise – for example, around understandings of confidentiality and privacy or whether the priority should be to care for or control service users (see Banks, 2004, pp. 125–148; Irvine *et al.*, 2002). There is also literature proposing ethical frameworks for how different professions should work together to create mutual respect and understanding (see Clark *et al.*, 2007); or proposing the development of new common professional values that integrate or supersede the specific ethical codes of individual professions (Bond, 1995).

How does a virtue-based approach to ethics help us in the context of this developing trend towards inter-professional working, specifically in relation to health and social care practice? The vignettes we use at the start of Chapters 4–10 are usually written in the voice of, and generally focus on the moral qualities of, one particular professional practitioner (either a health or a social care practitioner). Our focus is not on how practitioners from these different professions work together, nor on pointing out differences in the moral values (specifically virtues) of the different professionals. Our assumption is that the same key virtues are important for both health and social care professionals. Indeed, arguably the virtues we cover in this book are important for all human beings in leading a good life, and this includes professionals in a range of fields (from education to engineering). Some virtues (such as being caring) might be less likely to be included in a list of core virtues for engineers, while others not featured in our chapters might be regarded as more relevant (for example, honesty). However, our choice of virtues is relatively generic, and we would argue that all are equally relevant to practitioners in both the health and the social care fields.

By focusing on the virtues of the professional practitioner, rather than on ethical principles or rules of action, this gives a common starting point for professional ethics. We can agree, for example, that being caring is a valuable moral quality in health and social care professionals, while it will be developed and demonstrated in very different ways by people in different professional roles in different contexts. The context in which a professional is placed often contributes significantly to the way in which a particular virtue is demonstrated. The context is partly constituted by the nature of professional role (whether the protagonist is a nurse, midwife, paramedic, social worker or youth offending team manager) as well as by the other actors involved, the organisational context and other particular circumstances. The experienced nurse in Chapter 5, who very carefully worked with a woman to insert a naso-gastric tube, was demonstrating 'being caring' in a nursing context, combining professional skill with empathy and compassion. Nicola, the social worker from a hospice, who walked up the garden path to visit a man while envisioning what he might be thinking about the state of his life, was being caring in a completely different context, orienting herself as a potentially unwelcome visitor to the man's perspective and concerns. Interestingly, Nicola was accompanied on her visit by a nurse, with whom she shared her thoughts about what the man they were going to visit might be feeling and thinking. We would expect the nurse to appreciate these caring thoughts, as they would also be relevant to her role in this context.

Concluding comments

In a paper published in 1923, Mary Richmond, a pioneer of professional social work, discussed the character and contribution of founding nurse Florence Nightingale. Richmond was interested in the role of biography and its application to social work and was struck by similarities between the views and ideals of Nightingale and those prevailing in social work at that time. Richmond (1930, pp. 554–555) cites Nightingale's correspondence with Benjamin Jowett, Master of Balliol College, Oxford, who wrote as follows:

It is necessary for the safety of life that we should understand the characters of those among who[m] we are placed. But if we are only critical, or only capable of feeling pain at differences, then blind affection 'which covers a multitude of sins', is far better. It is useless to be intelligent if we see only the defects of others, and fail to recognise the good elements upon which we might work.

The role of character and the significance of what we are calling 'the virtues' was, in Richmond's time, well accepted. Although, as we discuss in Chapter 2 of this book, a virtue-based approach in the context of professional ethics has now been overtaken by principle-based approaches, character and virtue have been regarded as important in the caring professions since their inception. Richmond's paper suggests an early consideration of the possibility of shared ideals between nursing and social work, paving the way or beginning the quest, perhaps, for an inter-professional ethics.

Part of what we hope to achieve with this book is to create further opportunities for ethical dialogue between different professional practitioners working in the fields of health and social care. Irvine and McPhee (2007, p. 150) point out that much discussion relating to multiprofessional teams tends to focus on moral conflict. Yet the need is, rather, for a readiness to engage with each other in ethical dialogue, to articulate and justify ethical concerns and values. In virtue-based professional ethics, the concepts of professional roles, and the regulative ideals underpinning such roles, are very important. This entails having a concept of what it means to be a good social worker or a good nurse in a particular situation. Equally important is having an understanding of what it means to be a good professional (regardless of one's particular profession), and understanding and respecting the professional roles of others with whom one works. The roles of professionals in health and social care settings are frequently difficult – emotionally charged, potentially powerful, characterised by uncertainty and often constrained. Being a good enough practitioner is seldom easy. We hope that reading about and reflecting on examples from practitioners from a range of professional backgrounds in health and social care will raise questions, offer some insights, role models and contribute to the continual revisiting and reinvigorating that is constantly needed for the practice of ethics in professional life.

Selected lists of virtues

Aristotle (1992 edition) *Eudemian Ethics*	Bravery, endurance, temperance, justice, fair-mindedness, liberality, magnificence, friendliness, truthfulness, gentle temper, shame, dignity, pride, practical wisdom.
Aristotle (1976 edition) *Nicomachean Ethics*	Courage, temperance, liberality, magnificence, magnanimity, proper ambition, patience, truthfulness, wittiness, friendliness, modesty, righteous indignation.
Vidler (1964)	Justice, temperance, prudence, innocence, gentleness, chastity, modesty, piety, obedience, patriotism, felicity.
Geach (1977)	Courage, justice, temperance, prudence, faith, hope, charity.
Foot (1978)	Courage, justice, temperance, wisdom.
MacIntyre (1985)	Courage, justice, honesty.
Comte-Sponville (2002) *great virtues*	Courage, politeness, fidelity, prudence, temperance, justice, generosity, compassion, mercy, gratitude, humility, simplicity, tolerance, purity, gentleness, good faith, humour, love.

(Continued)

Carr (1991)	*Self-control* – courage, temperance, chastity. *Attachment* – unselfishness, sympathy, temperance, benevolence, considerateness, generosity, courtesy.
Fowler (1997) *nursing virtues*	Courage, benevolence, care, compassion, competence, devotion, faithfulness, honesty, integrity, justness, kindness, knowledgeable, loving, loyal, loyal, nonmalevolent, prudent, skilled, teachable, temperate, tolerate, trustworthy, wise, understanding, truthful.
Sellman (1997) *nursing virtues*	Obedience, punctuality, observation.
Rhodes (1986) *social work virtues*	Compassion, detached caring, warmth, honesty, moral courage, Hopefulness, humility.
Bowles et al (2006) *social work virtues*	Open-mindedness, practical reasoning, moral courage, reflectiveness/ critical reflection, empathy, integrity/commitment to social work values, discretion, tolerance/valuing diversity, good judgement/'wisdom'.
Oakley and Cocking (2001) *doctors' virtues*	Courage, beneficence, truthfulness, trustworthiness, humility.
Horner (2000) *public health virtues*	Courage, temperance, truthfulness, righteous indignation, patience modesty, friendliness, liberality.
Labacqz (1985) *patients' virtues*	Courage, patience, hope.

References

Adams, R. (2006) *A Theory of Virtue: Excellence in Being for the Good*, Oxford, Oxford University Press.

Adams, R., Dominelli, L., and Payne, M. (eds) (2005) *Social Work Futures: Crossing Boundaries, Transforming Practice*, Basingstoke, Palgrave Macmillan.

Airaksinen, T. (1994) 'Service and science in professional life', in R. Chadwick (ed.), *Ethics and the Professions*, Aldershot, Avebury, pp. 1–13.

Airaksinen, T. (1998) 'Professional ethics', in R. Chadwick (ed.), *Encyclopedia of Applied Ethics, Vol. 3*, San Diego, Academic Press, pp. 671–682.

Anscombe, E. (1958) 'Modern moral philosophy', *Philosophy*, vol. 33, pp. 1–19.

Aquinas, T. (1993 Edition) *Aquinas: Selected Philosophical Writings*, T. McDermott (ed.), Oxford, Oxford University Press.

Aristotle (1954 Edition) *The Nichomachean Ethics of Aristotle*, trans. Sir D. Ross, London, Oxford University Press.

Aristotle (1976 Edition) *The Ethics of Aristotle: The Nicomachean Ethics*, trans. J. Thomson, Introduction J. Barnes, London, Penguin Books.

Aristotle (1991 Edition) *The Art of Rhetoric*, London, Penguin Books.

Aristotle (1992 Edition) *Eudemian Ethics Books 1, 11 and V111,* Commentary by M. Woods, 2nd Edn, Oxford, Clarendon Press.

Armstrong, A. (2007) *Nursing Ethics: A Virtue-Based Approach*, Basingstoke, Palgrave Macmillan.

Atkins, S. and Murphy, K. (1994) 'Reflective practice', *Nursing Standard*, vol. 8, no. 39, pp. 256–260.

Audi, R. (1997) *Moral Knowledge and Ethical Character*, Oxford, Oxford University Press.

Australian Association of Social Workers (1999) *AASW Code of Ethics*, Kingston, AASW.

Baier, A. (1985) *Postures of the Mind: Essays on Mind and Morals*, Minneapolis, Minneapolis University Press.

Baier, A. (1986) 'Trust and anti-trust', *Ethics*, vol. 96, pp. 231–260.

Banks, S. (2003) 'The use of learning journals to encourage ethical reflection during fieldwork practice', in S. Banks and K. Nøhr (eds), *Teaching Practical Ethics for the Social Professions*, Copenhagen, FESET, pp. 53–67.

Banks, S. (2004) *Ethics, Accountability and the Social Professions*, Basingstoke, Palgrave Macmillan.

Banks, S. (2006) *Ethics and Values in Social Work*, 3rd Edn, Basingstoke, Palgrave Macmillan.

Banks, S. (2007) 'Becoming critical: developing the community practitioner', in H. Butcher, S. Banks, P. Henderson with J. Robertson, *Critical Community Practice*, Bristol, The Policy Press, pp. 133–152.

Barron, M. (1997) 'Kantian ethics', in M. Barron, P. Pettit, and M. Slote, *Three Methods of Ethics*, Oxford, Blackwell, pp. 1–91.

Bauby, J.-D. (1997) *The Diving-Bell and the Butterfly*, London, Fourth Estate Limited.

Beauchamp, T. (2003) 'The origins, goals, and core commitments of *The Belmont Report* and *Principles of Biomedical Ethics*', in J. Walter and E. Klein (eds), *The Story of Bioethics: From Seminal Works to Contemporary Explorations*, Washington DC, Georgetown University Press, pp. 17–46.

Beauchamp, T. and Childress, J. (1979) *Principles of Biomedical Ethics*, 1st Edn, Oxford and New York, Oxford University Press.

Beauchamp, T. and Childress, J. (1994) *Principles of Biomedical Ethics*, 4th Edn, Oxford and New York, Oxford University Press.

Beauchamp, T. and Childress, J. (2001) *Principles of Biomedical Ethics*, 5th Edn, Oxford and New York, Oxford University Press.

Beckett, C. and Maynard, A. (2005) *Values and Ethics in Social Work: An Introduction*, London, Sage.

Bellah, R., Masden, R., Sullivan, W., Swidler, A., and Tipton, S. (1988) *Habits of the Heart: Middle America Observed*, London, Century Hutchinson.

Bennett, A. (2005) *Untold Stories*, London, Faber and Faber.

Blackburn, S. (1999) *Think*, Oxford, Oxford University Press.

Blum, L. (1994) *Moral Perception and Particularity*, Cambridge, Cambridge University Press.

Bolsin, D. (2003) 'Whistleblowing: commentary', *Medical Education*, vol. 37, pp. 294–296

Bolsin, D., Patrick, A., Colson, M., Creatie, B., and Freestone, L. (2005) 'New technology to enable personal monitoring and incident reporting can transform professional culture: the potential to favourably impact the future of health care', *Journal of Evaluation in Clinical Practice*, vol. 11, no. 5, pp. 499–506.

Bond, T. (1995) *Confidentiality about HIV in Multidisciplinary Teams*, Newcastle, Northern and Yorkshire Regional Health Authority.

Boseley, S. (2001) 'Arrogance let babies die – now a chance to mend NHS', *The Guardian*, 19th July, p. 1.

Boss, J. (1998) *Ethics for Life: An Interdisciplinary and Multi-Cultural Introduction*, Mountain View, CA, Mayfield.

Boud, D. and Walker, D. (1998) 'Promoting reflection in professional courses: the challenge of context', *Studies in Higher Education*, vol. 23, no. 2, pp. 191–206.

Bowden, P. (1997) *Caring: Gender Sensitive Ethics*, London, Routledge.

Bowles, W., Collingridge, M., Curry, S., and Valentine, B. (2006) *Ethical Practice in Social Work: An Applied Approach*, Crow's Nest, New South Wales, Allen and Unwin.

Bradshaw, P. (1996) 'Yes! there is an ethics of care: an answer for Peter Allmark', *Journal of Medical Ethics*, vol. 22, pp. 8–12.

Brandt, R. (1976) 'The concept of welfare', in N. Timms and D. Watson (eds), *Talking about Welfare: Readings in Philosophy and Social Policy*, London, Routledge and Kegan Paul, pp. 64–87.

Briskman, L. (2005) 'Pushing ethical boundaries for children and families: confidentiality, transparency and transformation', in R. Adams, L. Dominelli, and M. Payne (eds), *Social Work Futures: Crossing Boundaries, Transforming Practice*, Basingstoke, Palgrave Macmillan, pp. 208–220.

British Association of Social Workers (1976) *A Code of Ethics for Social Work*, Birmingham, BASW.

British Association of Social Workers (2002) *The Code of Ethics for Social Work*, Birmingham, BASW.

Brown, G. (2007a) *Courage: Eight Portraits*, London, Bloomsbury.

Brown, G. (2007b) *Britain's Everyday Heroes*, Edinburgh, Mainstream Publishing Company.

Brykczyńska, G. (1997) 'A brief overview of the epistemology of caring', in G. Brykczyńska (ed.), *Caring: The Compassion and Wisdom of Nursing*, London, Arnold, pp. 1–9.

Butcher, H., Banks, S., Henderson, P. with Robertson, J. (2007) *Critical Community Practice*, Bristol, The Policy Press.

Calhoun, C. (1995) 'Standing for something', *Journal of Philosophy*, vol. 92, pp. 235–260.

Campbell, A. (2005) 'A virtue-ethics approach' in R. Ashcroft, A. Lucassen, M. Parker, M. Verkerk, and G. Widdershoven (eds), *Case Analysis in Clinical Ethics*, Cambridge, Cambridge University Press, pp. 45–56.

Carr, D. (1999) 'Professional education and professional ethics', *Journal of Applied Philosophy*, vol. 16, no. 1, pp. 33–46.

Carter, H. and Ward, D. (2002) 'Britain's worst serial killer: 215 dead but we still don't know why', *The Guardian*, 20th July.

Casey, J. (1990) *Pagan Virtue: An Essay in Ethics*, Oxford, Clarendon Press.

Chadwick, R. and Levitt, M. (1997) 'Professions in crisis: the ethical response', in J. Scally (ed.), *Ethics in Crisis?* Dublin, Veritas, pp. 55–65.

Chambliss, D. (1996) *Beyond Caring: Hospitals, Nurses and the Social Organisation of Ethics*, Chicago, University of Chicago Press.

Charleton, M. (2007) *Ethics for Social Care in Ireland: Philosophy and Practice*, Dublin, Gill and Macmillan.

Clark, C. (2000) *Social Work Ethics: Politics, Principles and Practice*, Basingstoke, Macmillan.

Clark, C. (2006), 'Moral character in social work', *British Journal of Social Work*, vol. 36, pp. 75–89.

Clark, P., Cott, C., and Drinka, T. (2007) 'Theory and practice in interprofessional ethics: a framework for understanding ethical issues in health care teams', *Journal of Interprofessional Care*, vol. 21, no. 6, pp. 591–603.

Clifford, D. (2002) 'Resolving uncertainties? The contribution of some recent feminist ethical theory to the social professions', *European Journal of Social Work*, vol. 5, no. 1, pp. 31–41.

Comte-Sponville, A. (2002) *A Short Treatise on the Great Virtues: The Uses of Philosophy in Everyday Life*, London, William Heinemann.

Comte-Sponville, A. (2003) *A Short Treatise on the Great Virtues: The Uses of Philosophy in Everyday Life*, London, Vintage.

Confucius (1979 Edition) *The Analects*, London, Penguin Books.

Cottingham, J. (1996) 'Partiality and the virtues', in R. Crisp (ed.), *How Should One Live? Essays on the Virtues*, Oxford, Oxford University Press, pp. 57–76.

Cox, D., La Caze, M., and Levine, M. (2003) *Integrity and the Fragile Self*, Aldershot, Ashgate.

Cox, D., La Caze, M., and Levine, M. (2005) 'Integrity', in E. Zalta (ed.), *Stanford Encyclopedia of Philosophy*, http://plato.stanford.edu/entries/integrity, accessed November 2005.

Cree, V. and Davis, A. (2007) *Social Work: Voices from the Inside*, London, Routledge.

Crisp, R. (ed.) (1996) *How Should One Live? Essays on the Virtues*, Oxford, Oxford University Press.

Crisp, R. and Slote, M. (1997a) 'Introduction', in R. Crisp and M. Slote (eds), *Virtue Ethics*, Oxford, Oxford University Press, pp. 1–25.

Crisp, R. and Slote, M. (eds) (1997b) *Virtue Ethics*, Oxford, Oxford University Press.

Daloz Parks, S. (1993) 'Professional ethics, moral courage, and the limits of personal virtue', in B. Darling-Smith (ed.), *Can Virtue Be Taught?* Notre Dame, University of Notre Dame Press.

Darley, J. and Batson, C. (1973) 'From Jerusalem to Jericho: a study of situational and dispositional variables in helping behaviour', *Journal of Personality and Social Psychology*, vol. 27, no. 1, pp. 100–108.

Darwell, S. (1995) 'Two kinds of respect', in R. Dillon (ed.), *Dignity, Character and Self-Respect*, London, Routledge.

Davies, C. (1998) 'Caregiving, carework and professional care', in A. Brechin, J. Walmsley, J. Katz, and S. Peace (eds), *Care Matters: Concepts, Practice and Research in Health and Social Care*, London, Sage, pp. 126–138.

De Raeve, L. (2006) 'Virtue ethics', in A. Davis, V. Tschudin, and L. De Raeve (eds), *Essentials of Teaching and Learning in Nursing Ethics*, London, Churchill Livingstone, Elsevier, pp. 97–108.

Devettere, R. (2002) *Introduction to Virtue Ethics: Insights of the Ancient Greeks*, Washington, Georgetown University Press.

Dickenson, D. (1994) 'Nurse time as a scarce health care resource', in G. Hunt (ed.), *Ethical Issues in Nursing*, London, Routledge, pp. 207–212.

Dillon, R. (2005) 'Respect', in E. Zalta (ed.),.*Stanford Encyclopaedia of Philosophy*, http://plato.stanford.edu/archives/win2005/entries/respect/, accessed May 2008.

Dobson, R. (1998) 'Sick to death of morals', *Independent*, 9th June, p. 12.

Dominelli, L. (2002) *Anti Oppressive Social Work Theory and Practice*, Basingstoke, Palgrave Macmillan.

Doris, J. (2002) *Lack of Character: Personality and Moral Behaviour*, Cambridge, Cambridge University Press.

Downie, R. and MacNaughton, J. (2000) *Clinical Judgement: Evidence in Practice*, Oxford, Oxford University Press.

Downie, R. and Telfer, E. (1980) *Caring and Curing*, London, Methuen.

Driver, J. (1996) 'The virtues and human nature', in R. Crisp (ed.), *How Should One Live? Essays on the Virtues*, Oxford, Oxford University Press, pp. 111–129.

Fish, D. and Coles, C. (1998) *Developing Professional Judgement in Health Care: Learning Through the Critical Appreciation of Practice*, London, Butterworth-Heinemann.

Foot, P. (1978) *Virtues and Vices and Other Essays in Moral Philosophy*, Oxford, Basil Blackwell.

Fowler, M. (1997) 'Nursing's ethics', in A. Davis, M. Aroskar, J. Liaschenko, and T. Drought (eds), *Ethical Dilemmas and Nursing Practice*, 4th Edn, Stamford, Appleton and Lange.

Frankfurt, H. (1987) 'Identification and wholeheartedness', in F. Schoeman (ed.), *Responsibility, Character, and the Emotions: New Essays in Moral Psychology*, New York, Cambridge University Press.

Frankl, V. (2004) *Man's Search for Meaning*, London, Rider.

Fraser, N. and Honneth, A. (2003) *Redistribution or Recognition: a Political-Philosophical Exchange*, London, Verso.

Freidson, E. (1983) 'The theory of the professions: state of the art', in R. Dingwall and P. Lewis (eds), *The Sociology of the Professions: Lawyers, Doctors and Others*, Basingstoke, Macmillian, pp. 19–37.

Fry, S. (1989) 'The role of caring in a theory of nursing ethics', *Hypatia*, vol. 4, no. 2, pp. 88–103.

Gallagher, A. (2003) *Healthcare Virtues and Professional Education,* Unpublished PhD, Preston, University of Central Lancashire.

Gallagher, A. (2004) 'Dignity and respect for dignity – two key professional values: implications for nursing practice', *Nursing Ethics*, vol. 11, no. 6, pp. 587–599.

Gallagher, A. (2007) 'The respectful nurse', *Nursing Ethics*, vol. 14, no. 3, pp. 360–371.

Gastmans, C. (2006) 'The care perspective in healthcare ethics', in A. Davis, V. Tschudin, and L. de Raeve (eds), *Essentials of Teaching and Learning in Nursing Ethics: Perspectives and Methods*, Edinburgh, Churchill Livingstone Elsevier, pp. 135–148.

Geach, P. (1977) *The Virtues: The Stanton Lectures 1973–4*, London, Cambridge University Press.

General Medical Council (2006) *Good Medical Practice: Duties of a Doctor*, London, GMC.

General Social Care Council (2004) *Code of Practice for Social Care Workers*, London, GSCC.

Giddens, A. (1990) *The Consequences of Modernity*, Stanford, Stanford University Press.

Gilligan, C. (1982) *In a Different Voice: Psychological Theory and Women's Development*, Cambridge, MA, Harvard University Press.

Gilligan, C. (1993) *In a Different Voice: Psychological Theory and Women's Development*, 2nd Edn, Cambridge, MA, Harvard University Press.

Goldie, P. (2000) *The Emotions: A Philosophical Exploration*, Oxford, Oxford University Press.

Goldie, P. (2004) *On Personality*, London, Routledge.

Goovaerts, H. (2003) 'Working with a staged plan', in S. Banks and K. Nøhr (eds), *Teaching Practical Ethics for the Social Professions*, Copenhagen, FESET, pp. 83–93.

Govier, T. (1997) *Social Trust and Human Communities*, Montreal and Kingston, McGill-Queen's University Press.

Graham, J. (2001) 'Does integrity require moral goodness?', *Ratio (new series)*, vol. XIV, pp. 234–251.

Hamilton, E. and Cairns, H. (eds) (1961) *The Collected Dialogues of Plato*, New York, Pantheon Books.

Hanford, L. (1994) 'Nursing and the concept of care: an appraisal of noddings' theory', in G. Hunt (ed.), *Ethical Issues in Nursing*, London, Routledge, pp. 181–197.

Hardcastle, D., Powers, P., and Wencour, S. (2004) *Community Practice: Theories and Skills for Social Workers*, 2nd Edn, New York, Oxford University Press.

Harding Clark, M. (2006) *The Lourdes Hospital Inquiry – An Inquiry into Peripartum Hysterectomy at Our Lady of Lourdes Hospital, Drogheda*, Dublin, The Stationery Office.

Hardingham, L. (2004) 'Integrity and moral residue: nurses as participants in a moral community', *Nursing Philosophy*, vol. 5, pp.127–134.

Harman, G. (1999) 'Moral philosophy meets social psychology: virtue ethics and the fundamental attribution error', *Proceedings of the Aristotelian Society*, vol. 99, pp. 315–331.

Harper, D. (2001) *Online Etymology Dictionary*, http://www.etymonline.com/index. php?term=character, accessed May 2008.

Hekman, S. (1995) *Moral Voices, Moral Selves: Carol Gilligan and Feminist Moral Theory*, Cambridge, Polity Press.

Held, V. (2006) *The Ethics of Care: Personal, Political, and Global*, Oxford, Oxford University Press.

Hochschild, A. (1983) *The Managed Heart: Commercialisation of Human Feeling*, Berkeley, University of California Press.

Hoggett, P., Beedell, P., Jimenez, L., Mayo, M., and Miller, C. (2006) 'Identity, life history and commitment to welfare', *Journal of Social Policy*, vol. 35, no. 4, pp. 689–704.

Honneth, A. (2001) 'Recognition or redistribution? Changing perspectives on the moral order of society', *Theory, Culture & Society*, vol. 18, no. 2–3, pp. 43–55.

Hope, A. and Timmel, S. (1999) *Training for Transformation: A Handbook for Community Workers (book 4)*, London, ITDG publishing.

Horner, S. (2000) 'For debate: the virtuous public health physician', *Journal of Public Health Medicine*, vol. 22, no. 1, pp. 48–53.

Horsburgh, H. (1960) 'The ethics of trust', *Philosophical Quarterly*, vol. 10, pp. 343–354.

Hughes, G. (2001) *Aristotle on Ethics*, London, Routledge.

Hugman, R. (2005) *New Approaches in Ethics for the Caring Professions*, Basingstoke and New York, Palgrave Macmillan.

Hume, D. (1739/1960) *A Treatise of Human Nature*, edited by L. Selby-Bigge, Oxford, Clarendon Press.

Humphreys, J. (2005) *The Story of Virtue: Universal Lessons on How to Live*, Dublin, The Liffey Press.

Hunt, G. (ed.) (1998) *Whistleblowing in the Social Services: Public Accountability and Professional Practice*, London, Arnold.

Hursthouse, R. (1987) *Beginning Lives*, Oxford, Blackwell in association with the Open University.

Hursthouse, R. (1991) 'Virtue theory and abortion', *Philosophy and Public Affairs*, vol. 20, no. 3, pp. 223–246.

Hursthouse, R. (1999) *On Virtue Ethics*, Oxford, Oxford University Press.

Hymes, D. (1981) *'In vain I tried to tell you'. Essays in Native American Ethnopoetics*, Philadelphia, University of Pennsylvania Press.

International Council of Nurses (2008) *Definition of Nursing*, Geneva, ICN, www.icn.ch/definition.htm, accessed April 2008.

International Federation of Social Workers (2000) *Definition of Social Work*, www.ifsw.org/en/p38000208.html, accessed April 2008.

Irvine, R. and McPhee, J. (2007) 'Multidisciplinary team practice in law and ethics: an Australian perspective' in A. Leathard and S. McLaren (eds), *Ethics: Contemporary Challenges in Health and Social Care*, Bristol, The Policy Press, pp. 143–155.

Irvine, R., Kerridge, I., McPhee, J., and Freeman, S. (2002) 'Interprofessionalism and ethics: consensus or clash of cultures', *Journal of Interprofessional Care*, vol. 16, no. 3, pp. 199–210.

James, N. (1989) 'Emotional labour, skills and work in the social regulation of feeling', *The Sociological Review*, vol. 37, no. 1, pp. 15–42.

Johnson, T. (1972) *Professions and Power*, London, Macmillan.

Johnstone, M-J. (2004) *Bioethics: A Nursing Perspective,* 4th Edn, Sydney, Churchill Livingstone.

Kant, I. (1785/1964) *Groundwork of the Metaphysics of Morals*, trans. H. Paton, New York, Harper and Row.

Kant, I. (1797/1964) *The Doctrine of Virtue*, trans. M. Gregor, New York, Harper and Row.

Kekes, J. (1993) *The Morality of Pluralism*, Princeton, Princeton University Press.

Kennedy, I. (2001) *Bristol Royal Infirmary Report,* http://www.bristol-inquiry.org.uk/final_report/report/Summary.htm, accessed January 2008.

Kittay, E. (1999) *Love's Labour: Essays on women, Equality, and Dependency*, New York, Harper and Row.

Koehn, D. (1994) *The Ground of Professional Ethics*, London, Routledge.

Kohlberg, L. (1981) *Essays on Moral Development: Volume 1, The Philosophy of Moral Development: Moral Stages and the Idea of Justice*, New York, Harper and Row.

Kohlberg, L. (1984) *Essays on Moral Development: Volume 2, The Psychology of Moral Development*, San Francisco, Harper and Row.

Kosman, L. (1999) 'Being properly affected: Virtues and feelings in Aristotle's ethics', in N. Sherman (ed.) *Aristotle's Ethics: Critical Essays*, Lanham, Rowman & Littlefield, pp. 261–276.

Kronman, A. (1987) 'Practical wisdom and professional character', *Social Philosophy and Policy*, vol. 4, no. 1, pp. 203–234.

Kupperman, J. (1990) *Character*, Oxford, Oxford University Press.

Labacqz, K. (1985) 'The virtuous patient', in E. Shelp (ed.), *Virtue and Medicine*, Dordrecht, D. Reidel Publishing Company, pp 278–288.

Laming, H. (2003) *The Victoria Climbié Inquiry*, London, The Stationery Office.

Langen, R. (2003) 'Exploring aspects of ethical theory through drama', in S. Banks and K. Nøhr (eds), *Teaching Practical Ethics for the Social Professions*, Copenhagen, FESET, pp. 107–122.

Liaschenko, J. (1994) 'Making a bridge: the moral work with patients we do not like', *Journal of Palliative Care*, vol. 3, no. 19, pp. 83–89.

Louden, R. (1998) 'Virtue ethics', in R. Chadwick (ed.), *Encyclopaedia of Applied Ethics, Vol. 4*, San Diego, Academic Press, pp. 491–498.

Luhmann, N. (1979) *Trust and Power*, New York, John Wiley and Sons.

Luhmann, N. (1988) 'Familiarity, confidence, trust: problems and perspectives', in D. Gambetta (ed.), *Trust: Making and Breaking Cooperative Relations*, Oxford, Blackwell.

Machin, S. (1998) 'Swimming against the tide: a social worker's experience of a secure hospital', in G. Hunt (ed.), *Whistleblowing in the Social Services: Public Accountability and Professional Practice*, London, Arnold, pp. 116–130.

MacIntyre, A. (1985) *After Virtue: A Study in Moral Theory*, 2nd Edn, London, Gerald Duckworth and Co. Ltd.

MacIntyre, A. (1999) *Dependent Rational Animals: Why Human Beings Need the Virtues*, London, Gerald Duckworth and Co. Ltd.

Marshall, T. (1976) 'The right to welfare', in N. Timms and D. Watson (eds), *Talking about Welfare: Readings in Philosophy and Social Policy*, London, Routledge and Kegan Paul, pp. 51–63.

Mason, A. (1996) 'MacIntyre on modernity and how it has marginalised the virtues', in R. Crisp (ed.), *How Should One Live?* Oxford, Oxford University Press, pp. 191–210.

McAuliffe, D. and Chenowith, L. (2008) 'Leave No stone unturned: the inclusive model of ethical decision-making', *Ethics and Social Welfare*, vol. 2, no. 1, pp 38–49.

McBeath, G. and Webb, S. (2002) 'Virtue ethics and social work: being lucky, realistic, and not doing one's duty', *British Journal of Social Work*, vol. 32, pp. 1015–1036.

McCarthy, J. and Deady, R. (2008) 'Moral distress reconsidered', *Nursing Ethics*, vol. 15, no. 2, pp. 254–262.

McDowell, J. (1997) 'Virtue and reason', in R. Crisp and M. Slote (eds), *Virtue Ethics*, Oxford, Oxford University Press, pp. 141–162.

McLaren, M. (2001) 'Feminist ethics: care as a virtue', in P. DesAutels and J. Waugh (eds), *Feminists Doing Ethics*, Lanham, Maryland, Rowman and Littlefield, pp. 101–117.

McLeod, C. (2006) 'Trust', in E. Zalta (ed.), *Stanford Encyclopedia of Philosophy*, www.plato.stanford.edu/entries/trust, accessed July 2007.

MENCAP (2007) *Death by Indifference*, London, MENCAP.

Merritt, M. (2000) 'Virtue ethics and situationist personality psychology', *Ethical Theory and Moral Practice*, vol. 3, pp. 365–383.

Middleton, D. (2006) 'Three types of self-respect', *Res Publica*, vol. 12, pp. 59–76.

Milgram, S. (1974) *Obedience to Authority*, New York, Harper and Row.

Mill, J.S. (1972) *Utilitarianism, On Liberty, and Considerations on Representative Government*, London, Dent.

Miller, D. (1994) 'Virtues, practices and justice', in J. Horton and S. Mendus (eds), *After MacIntyre*, Cambridge, Polity Press, pp. 245–264.

Montgomery Hunter, K., Charon, R., and Coulehan, J. (1995) 'The study of literature in medical education', *Academic Medicine*, vol. 70, no. 9, pp. 787–791.

Morrison, P. (1997) 'Patients' experiences of being cared for', in G. Brykczyńska (ed.), *Caring: The Compassion and Wisdom of Nursing*, London, Arnold, pp. 102–130.

Morse, J., Bottoroff, J., Neander, W., and Solberg, S. (1991) 'Comparative analysis of conceptualisations and theories of caring', *Image: Journal of Nursing Scholarship*, vol. 23, pp. 119–126.

Murdoch, I. (1970) *The Sovereignty of Good,* London, Routledge.

Musschenga, A. (2001) 'Education for moral integrity', *Journal of Philosophy of Education*, vol. 35, no. 2, pp. 219–235.

Nagel, T. (1979) 'The fragmentation of value', in T. Nagel, *Mortal Questions*, Cambridge, Cambridge University Press, pp. 128–141.

Nagel, T. (1980) 'Aristotle on eudaimonia', in A. Rorty, *Essays on Aristotle's Ethics,* Berkeley, University of California Press.

National Association of Social Workers (1999) *Code of Ethics*, Washington, NASW.

Noddings, N. (1984) *Caring: A Feminine Approach to Ethics and Moral Education*, Berkeley and Los Angeles, University of California Press.

Noddings, N. (2002) *Starting at Home: Caring and Social Policy*, Berkeley and Los Angeles, University of California Press.

Nozick, R. (1974) *Anarchy, State and Utopia*, Oxford, Blackwell.

Nursing and Midwifery Council (NMC) (2002) *Code of Professional Conduct*, London, NMC.

Nursing and Midwifery Council (NMC) (2004) *Fitness to Practise: Annual Report 2003–4*, London, NMC.

Nursing and Midwifery Council (NMC) (2008) *The Code: Standards of Conduct, Performance and Ethics for Nurses and Midwives*, London, NMC.

Nussbaum, M. (1990) *Love's Knowledge: Essays on Philosophy and Literature,* New York, Oxford University Press.

Nussbaum, M. (2000) *Women and Human Development*, Cambridge, Cambridge University Press.

Nussbaum, M. (2001) *Upheavals of Thought: The Intelligence of Emotions*, Cambridge, Cambridge University Press.

Nussbaum, M. (2004) *Hiding from Humanity: Disgust, Shame and the Law,* Princeton, Princeton University Press.

Nussbaum, M. (2006) *Frontiers of Justice*, Cambridge, Mass, Belnap/Harvard University Press.

Oakley, J. (1992) *Morality and the Emotions*, London, Routledge.

Oakley, J. and Cocking, D. (2001) *Virtue Ethics and Professional Roles*, Cambridge, Cambridge University Press.

Okin, S. (1994) 'Gender inequality and cultural difference', *Political Theory*, vol. 22, pp. 5–24.

O'Neill, O. (1996a) 'Kant's virtues', in R. Crisp (ed.), *How Should One Live: Essays on the Virtues*, Oxford, Oxford University Press, pp. 77–98.

O'Neill, O. (1996b) *Towards Justice and Virtue: A Constructive Account of Practical Reasoning*, Cambridge, Cambridge University Press.

O'Neill, O. (2002) *A Question of Trust*, Cambridge, Cambridge University Press.

Parton, N. (2003) 'Rethinking *professional* practice: the contributions of social constructionism and the feminist "ethics of care"', *British Journal of Social Work*, vol. 33, pp. 1–16.

Payne, M. (2000) 'Social work', in M. Davies (ed.), *Blackwell Encyclopedia of Social Work*, Oxford, Blackwell, p. 225.

Pellegrino, E. (1995) 'Toward a virtue-based normative ethics for the health professions', *Kennedy Institute of Ethics Journal*, vol. 3, no. 3, pp. 253–277.

Pellegrino, E. and Thomasma, D. (1981) *The Philosophical Basis of Medical Practice*, New York, Oxford University Press.

Pellegrino, E. and Thomasma, D. (1988) *For the Patient's Good: The Restoration of Beneficence in Health Care*, New York, Oxford University Press.

Pellegrino, E. and Thomasma, D. (1993) *The Virtues in Medical Practice*, New York, Oxford University Press.

Philippart, F. (2003) 'Using Socratic dialogue', in S. Banks and K. Nøhr (eds), *Teaching Practical Ethics for the Social Professions*, Copenhagen, FESET, pp. 69–82.

Phillips, C. (2004) *Six Questions of Socrates: A Modern-Day Journey of Discovery through World Philosophy*, New York, W.W. Norton and Co.

Pink, G. (1994) 'The price of truth', *British Medical Journal,* vol. 309, no. 6970, pp. 1700–1705.

Pithouse, A. and Atkinson, P. (1988) 'Telling the case: occupational narrative in a social work office', in N. Coupland (ed.), *Styles of Discourse*, London, Croom Helm, pp. 183–200.

Plato (1955) *The Republic*, trans. H. Lee, Harmondsworth, Penguin.

Potter, N. (2002) *How Can I be Trusted? A Virtue Theory of Trustworthiness*, Lanham, Maryland, Rowman and Littlefield.

Rafferty, A. (1996) *The Politics of Nursing Knowledge,* London, Routledge.

Rawls, J. (1971) *A Theory of Justice,* Oxford, Oxford University Press.

Rawls, J. (1973) *A Theory of Justice*, Oxford, Oxford University Press Paperback.

Rawls, J. (1993) *Political Liberalism*, New York, Columbia University Press.

Ray, S. (2006) 'Whistleblowing and organisational ethics', *Nursing Ethics*, vol. 13, pp. 438–445.

Raz, J. (2001) *Value, Respect and Attachment,* Cambridge, Cambridge University Press.

Reamer, F. (1999) *Social Work Values and Ethics*, 2nd Edn, New York, Columbia University Press.

Reiser, S. (1994) 'The ethical life of health care organizations', *The Hastings Center Report,* vol. 24, no. 6, pp. 28–34.

Rest, J. (1994) 'Background: theory and research', in J. Rest and D. Narváez (eds), *Moral Development in the Professions: Psychology and Applied Ethics*, Hillsdale, New Jersey, Lawrence Erlbaum Associates, pp. 1–26.

Rhodes, M. (1986) *Ethical Dilemmas in Social Work Practice*, Boston, Mass., Routledge and Kegan Paul.

Richmond, M. (1930) *The Long View: Papers and Addresses*, New York, Russell Sage Foundation.

Ricoeur, P. (2007) *Reflections on the Just*, trans. D. Pellauer, Chicago, University of Chicago Press.

Rolfe, G., Freshwater, D., and Jasper, M. (2001) *Critical Reflection for Nursing and the Helping Professions: A User's Guide*, Basingstoke, Palgrave Macmillan.

Ross, L. and Nisbet, R. (1991) *The Person and the Situation: Perspectives of Social Psychology*, New York, McGraw-Hill.

Rossiter, A., Prilleltensky, I., and Walsh-Bowers, R. (2000) 'A postmodern perspective on professional ethics', in B. Fawcett, B. Featherstone, J. Fook, and A. Rossiter (eds), *Postmodern Feminist Perspectives: Practice and Research in Social Work*, London, Routledge, pp. 83–103.

Royal College of Nursing (RCN) (1992) *The Value of Nursing*, London, RCN.

Royal College of Nursing (RCN) (2003) *Defining Nursing*, London, RCN.

Royal College of Nursing (RCN) (2008) *Defending Dignity – Challenges and Opportunities for Nursing*, London, RCN.

Ryle, G. (1949/1973) *The Concept of Mind*, London, Penguin.

Sammons, K. and Sherzer, J. (eds) (2000) *Translating Native American Verbal Art: Ethnopoetics and Ethnography of Speaking*, Smithsonian Institution Press, Washington.

Sandel, M. (1998) *Liberalism and the Limits of Justice*, 2nd Edn, Cambridge, Cambridge University Press.

Schneewind, J. (1997) 'The misfortunes of virtue', in R. Crisp and M. Slote (eds), *Virtue Ethics*, Oxford, Oxford University Press, pp. 178–200.

Schön, D. (1983) *The Reflective Practitioner: How Professionals Think in Action*, New York, Basic Books.

Schön, D. (1987) *Educating the Reflective Practitioner*, San Francisco, Jossey-Bass Publishers.

Scott, A. (1995) 'Aristotle, nursing and health care ethics' *Nursing Ethics*, vol. 2, no. 4, pp. 279–285.

Scott, A. (1996) 'Ethics education and nursing practice', *Nursing Ethics*, vol. 3, no. 1, pp. 54–63.

Scott, P. (2000) 'The relationship between the arts and medicine', *Journal of Medical Ethics: Medical Humanities*, vol. 26, no. 1, pp. 3–8.

Scott, P. (2003) 'Virtue, nursing and the moral domain of practice', in V. Tschudin (ed.), *Approaches to Ethics: Nursing Beyond Boundaries*, London, Butterworth-Heinemann, pp. 25–32.

Seligman, A. (1997) *The Problem of Trust*, Princeton, Princeton University Press.

Sellman, D. (1997) 'The virtues in the moral education of nurses: Florence Nightingale revisited' *Nursing Ethics*, vol. 4, no. 1, pp. 3–11.

Sellman, D. (2005) 'Towards an understanding of nursing as a response to human vulnerability' *Nursing Philosophy*, vol. 6, no. 1, pp. 2–10.

Sen, A. (1993) 'Capability and well-being', in M. Nussbaum and A. Sen (eds), *The Quality of Life*, Oxford, Clarendon Press, pp. 30–53.

Senge, P. (2006) *The Fifth Discipline: The Art and Practice of the Learning Organisation*, New York, Doubleday.

Shelp, E. (ed.) (1985) *Virtue and Medicine*, Dordrecht, D. Reidal Publishing Company.

Sherman, N. (ed.) (1999) 'The habituation of character', *Aristotle's Ethics: Critical Essays*, Lanham, Maryland, Rowman & Littlefield, pp. 231–260.

Simpson, P. (1977) 'Contemporary virtue ethics and Aristotle', in D. Statman (ed.), *Virtue Ethics: A Critical Reader*, Edinburgh, Edinburgh University Press, pp. 245–259.

Siegrist, H. (1994) 'The professions, state and government in theory and history', in T. Becher (ed.), *Governments and Professional Education*, Buckingham, SRHE and Open University Press, pp. 3–20.

Slote, M. (1995) *From Morality to Virtue*, Oxford, Oxford University Press.

Slote, M. (1997) 'Virtue ethics', in M. Barron, P. Pettit, and M. Slote, *Three Methods of Ethics*, Oxford, Blackwell, pp. 175–238.

Slote, M. (2000) 'Virtue ethics', in H. LaFollette (ed.), *The Blackwell Guide to Ethical Theory*, Oxford, Blackwell, pp. 325–347.

Slote, M. (2001) *Morals from Motives*, Oxford, Oxford University Press.

Slote, M. (2002) 'Justice as a virtue', in E. Zalta (ed.), *Stanford Encyclopedia of Philosophy*, http://plato.stanford.edu/entries/justice-virtue, accessed August 2007.

Slote, M. (2007) *The Ethics of Care and Empathy*, London, Routledge.

Smith, P. (1992) *The Emotional Labour of Nursing: how Nurses Care*, Basingstoke, MacMillan.

Smith, P. and Gray, B. (2001) 'Reassessing the concept of emotional labour in student nurse education: role of link lecturers and mentors in a time of change', *Nurse Education Today*, vol. 21, pp. 230–237.

Statman, D. (ed.) (1997a) 'Introduction to virtue ethics', *Virtue Ethics: A Critical Reader*, Edinburgh, Edinburgh University Press, pp. 3–41.

Statman, D. (ed.) (1997b) *Virtue Ethics: A Critical Reader*, Edinburgh, Edinburgh University Press.

Stempsey, W. (2004) 'Guilt, shame and medicine', in M. Evans, P. Louhiala, and R. Puustinen (eds), *Philosophy for Medicine: Applications in a Clinical Context*, Oxford, Radcliffe Medical Press, pp. 47–63.

Stocker, M. (1976) 'The schizophrenia of modern ethical theories', *The Journal of Philosophy*, vol. 73, no. 14, pp. 453–466.

Sundin-Huard, D. and Fahy, K. (1999) 'Moral distress, advocacy and burnout: theorising the relationships,' *International Journal of Nursing Practice*, vol. 5, pp. 8–13.

Swanton, C. (2003) *Virtue Ethics: A Pluralistic View*, Oxford, Oxford University Press.

Taylor, C. and White, S. (2000) *Practising Reflexivity in Health and Welfare*, Buckingham, Open University Press.

Taylor, G. and Wolfram, S. (1968) 'The self-regarding and other-regarding virtues', *The Philosophical Quarterly*, vol. 18, pp. 238–248.

Tessman, L. (2001) 'Critical virtue ethics: understanding oppression as morally damaging', in P. DesAutels and J. Waugh (eds), *Feminists Doing Ethics*, Lanham, Maryland, Rowman and Littlefield, pp. 79–100.

Tessman, L. (2005) *Burdened Virtues: Virtue Ethics for Liberatory Struggles*, Oxford, Oxford University Press.

The Shipman Inquiry, http://www.the-shipman-inquiry.org.uk, accessed April 2008.

Thompson, I., Melia, K., and Boyd, K. (2000) *Nursing Ethics*, 4th Edn, Edinburgh, Churchill Livingstone.

Thurgood, M. (2004) 'Engaging clients in their care and treatment', in I. Norman and I. Ryrie (eds), *The Art and Science of Mental Health Nursing*, Maidenhead, Open University Press.

Timmons, M. (2002) *Moral Theory: An Introduction*, Lanham, Maryland, Rowman and Littlefield.

Toon, P. (1993) 'After bioethics and towards virtue?' *Journal of Medical Ethics*, vol. 19, pp. 17–18.

Toon, P. (1999) *Towards a Philosophy of General Practice: A Study of the Virtuous Practitioner*, London, The Royal College of General Practitioners.

Tronto, J. (1993) *Moral Boundaries: A Political Argument for an Ethic of Care*, London, Routledge.

Tschudin, V. (2003) *Ethics in Nursing: The Caring Relationship*, Heinemann, Edinburgh.

Values Exchange, www.values-exchange.com, accessed May 2008.

Van Hooft, S. (2006a) *Understanding Virtue Ethics*, Chesham, Acumen.

Van Hooft, S. (2006b) *Caring About Health*, Aldershot, Ashgate.

Veatch, R. (1981) *A Theory of Medical Ethics*, New York, Basic Books.

Vetlesen, A. (1994) *Perception, Empathy and Judgment: An Inquiry into the Preconditions of Moral Performance*, University Park, Pennsylvania, The Pennsylvania State University Press.

Vidler, A. (1964) *Traditional Virtues Reassessed*, London, S.P.C.K.

Walker, M. (1998) *Moral Understandings: A Feminist Study in Ethics*, New York, Routledge.

Walker, M. (2006) *Moral Repair: Reconstructing Moral Relations after Wrongdoing*, Cambridge, Cambridge University Press.

Walzer, M. (1983) *Spheres of Justice*, New York, Basic Books.

Webster, G. and Baylis, F. (2000) 'Moral residue' in S. Rubin and L. Zoloth (eds), *Margin of Error: The Ethics of Mistakes in the Practice of Medicine*, Hagerstown, University Publishing Group, pp. 217–300.

White, S. and Stancombe, J. (2003) *Clinical Judgement in the Health and Welfare Professions: Extending the Evidence Base*, Maidenhead, Open University Press.

White, S., Fook, J., and Gardner, F. (eds) (2006) *Critical Reflection in Health and Social Care*, Maidenhead, Open University Press.

Williams, B. (1973) 'Integrity', in B. Williams and J. Smart, *Utilitarianism: For and Against*, Cambridge, Cambridge University Press, pp. 108–118.

Williams, B. (1981) 'Persons, character and morality', in B. Williams, *Moral Luck: Philosophical Papers 1973–1980*, Cambridge, Cambridge University Press, pp. 1–19.

Williams, B. (1985) *Ethics and the Limits of Philosophy*, London, Fontana Paperbacks and William Collins.

Williams, F. (2000) 'Principles of recognition and respect in welfare', in G. Lewis, S. Gewirtz, and J. Clarke (eds), *Rethinking Social Policy*, London, Sage, pp. 339–352.

Zimbardo, P. (2007) *The Lucifer Effect: How Good People Turn Evil*, London, Rider.

Author index

Subject index